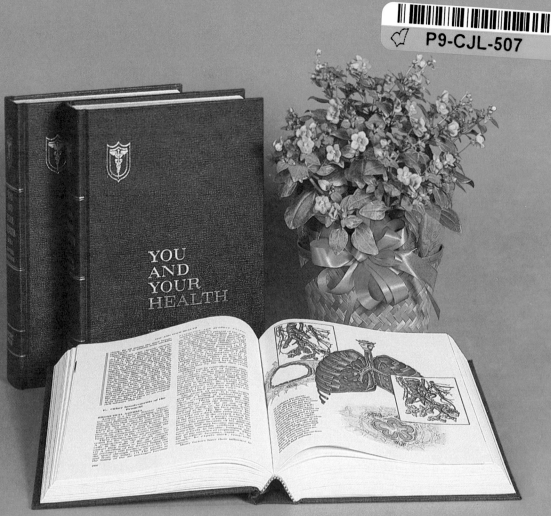

# Here's what the YOU AND YOUR HEALTH Medical Set can do for you.

- Puts the medical advice of 30 specialists at your fingertips.
- Shows you how to have a better life.
- Provides you with hundreds of practical tips for successful family raising.
- Explains, in easy-to-understand language, the symptoms of many common diseases.
- Gives you important lifesaving, first-aid tips.
- Supplies you with a number of simple, yet effective, home treatments.
- Illustrates the topics with hundreds of photos and drawings.
- Lists symptoms that will help you determine if a physician's help is needed.
- Clearly explains the basics of proper nutrition. Sample menus also included.
- Includes a useful section in volume 1 where you can record your family's medical history.

# VOLUME 1
New Edition

# You and Your Health

## More Abundant Living

## In three volumes, illustrated

Harold Shryock, M.A., M.D., and
Mervyn G. Hardinge, M.D.,
Dr.P.H., Ph.D.

In Collaboration With 28 Leading Medical Specialists

Published jointly by

**PACIFIC PRESS PUBLISHING ASSOCIATION**
Boise, ID 83707
Oshawa, Ontario, Canada

**REVIEW AND HERALD PUBLISHING ASSOCIATION**
Washington, DC 20039-0555
Hagerstown, MD 21740

ISBN 0-8163-0533-1

88 89 90 ● 6 5

# Collaborating Specialists

These volumes, covering a broad spectrum of health and medical topics, are published in collaboration with specialists who have checked material pertaining to their fields and contributed relevant information. Acknowledgment is due to the following teachers on the faculties of Loma Linda University, Loma Linda, California, and to others as identified.

R. Richards Banks, Ph.D., Licensed Psychologist
Jeffrey D. Cao, M.D., Assistant Professor of Pathology
C. Raymond Cress, Ph.D., Associate Professor of Pharmacology
Clarence W. Dail, M.D., Professor of Internal Medicine and Physical Medicine
Glenn L. Foster, M.D., Professor of Internal Medicine (Cardiology)
Herald A. Habenicht, M.D., Associate Professor of Health Education, Andrews University, Berrien Springs, Michigan
Henry L. Hadley, M.D., Professor of Urology
Richard H. Hart, M.D., Dr. P.H., Assistant Professor of Internal Medicine
Gustave H. Hoehn, M.D., Associate Clinical Professor of Internal Medicine (Dermatology)
Guy M. Hunt, M.D., M.S., Professor of Anatomy and Internal Medicine (Neurology)
Marion K. Jones, M.D., Psychiatric Service, Reading Institute of Rehabilitation, Reading, Pennsylvania
James D. Kettering, Ph.D., Associate Professor of Microbiology
Edwin H. Krick, M.D., M.P.H., Associate Professor of Internal Medicine
Irvin N. Kuhn, M.D., Professor of Internal Medicine
Benjamin H. S. Lau, M.D., Ph.D., Associate Professor of Microbiology
James I. McNeill, M.D., Professor of Ophthalmology
J. Lamont Murdoch, M.D., Professor of Internal Medicine (Endocrinology)
Robert L. Nutter, Ph.D., Professor of Microbiology
U. D. Register, Ph.D., Professor of Biochemistry and Nutrition
James A. Sadoyama, M.D., Associate Clinical Professor of Otolaryngology
Elmer P. Sakala, M.D., Assistant Professor of Gynecology and Obstetrics

Edwin F. Shryock, D.D.S., M.S., Associate Professor of Restorative Dentistry

George T. Simpson, Ed.D., Professor Emeritus of Counselor Education

Carrol S. Small, M.D., Professor of Pathology

Marilyn Christian Smith, Ed.D., Professor of Nursing

Edward D. Wagner, Ph.D., Professor of Microbiology

G. Carleton Wallace, M.D., Associate Clinical Professor of Orthopedic Surgery

Raymond O. West, M.D., M.P.H., Professor of Family Medicine and Epidemiology

# CONTENTS

# Volume 1—More Abundant Living

SECTION I—Dimensions of Life

  1. Life Has Length, Breadth, and Depth     15

SECTION II—The Perpetuation of Life

  2. Both Parents Contribute     23
  3. Motherhood in Prospect     29
  4. The Child's Development Before Birth     44
  5. Childbirth     53
  6. Care of the Infant: in Health, in Illness     61
  7. Patterns of Growth and Development     81

SECTION III—On Being Good Parents

  8. The Philosophy of Parenthood     93
  9. The Father's Part     101
  10. The Child's Need for Love     107
  11. Play Activities     112
  12. Discussing Intimate Matters     117
  13. Preparing the Child for Life     124
  14. Hazards of Homelife     132
  15. The Home's Regulations     143
  16. Educational and Vocational Guidance     154
  17. A Child's Problems and Illnesses     162

SECTION IV—On the Threshold of Adulthood

  18. A New Individuality     211
  19. Entering Adulthood     215
  20. Facing Life's Challenges     224
  21. Relationships With Parents Must Change     230
  22. Learning to Be Friendly     235

SECTION V—The Teenager

  23. The Urge to Experiment     241
  24. How Soon to Love?     246
  25. Petting, Pregnancy Too Soon, Homosexuality     251
  26. Teens' Health, Health Problems, and Hazards     258
  27. Teenage Financing     272

SECTION VI—Courtship and Marriage

  28. Problems of Courtship     279
  29. On Getting Married     285

SECTION VII—Husband and Wife

30. Respecting Each Other                           297
31. Differences in Belief                           304
32. Handling the Money                              309
33. Dealing With the Children                       315
34. The Intimate Side of Marriage                   320
35. Reasons for Tensions                            331
36. Finding the Trouble                             339
37. Rising Above Mistakes                           347
38. Avoiding Divorce                                351

SECTION VIII—Middle and Later Life

39. Adjusting to Retirement                         359
40. Illness During Later Life                       366
41. When Vigor Declines                             374

SECTION IX—Keynotes for Abundant Living

42. The Tone of Success                             381
43. The Foundations of Happiness                    385
44. Personal Maturity                               390
45. The Knack of Getting Along With People          398
46. Rising Above Moodiness                          406
47. The Control of Temper                           412
48. Imagination as an Ally                          418
49. Facing Reality                                  424
50. Mentality: Your Great Asset                     429

SECTION X—Safeguards to Health

51. Protecting Community Health                     447
52. Fitness                                         461
53. Choice of Food                                  476
54. Personal Indulgences                            490
55. Drugs: Good and Bad                             513

FAMILY MEDICAL RECORDS                              538

GENERAL INDEX                                       557

# Volume 2—The Human Body; Diseases; Symptoms

SECTION I—Combating Disease

Progress in Medicine — What Your Doctor Can Do for You — Helps for Diagnosis — Why Disease?

SECTION II—The Body's Defenses; Symptoms

The Marvelous Body and Its Defenses — Common Problems and Symptoms

SECTION III—The Heart; Circulatory Systems

The Heart, Blood Vessels, and Blood — Diseases of the Heart — Cardiovascular Disorders; Blood Vessel Diseases — Blood Diseases — The Lymphoid System and Related Diseases

SECTION IV—The Respiratory System

The Larynx, Air Passages, and Lungs — Diseases of the Respiratory Organs

SECTION V—The Digestive System

The Mouth and Teeth — Problems of the Mouth and Teeth — The Stomach and Intestines — Diseases of the Digestive Organs — The Liver, Gallbladder, and Pancreas — Diseases of the Liver, Gallbladder, and Pancreas

SECTION VI—The Skeletal System

The Body's Framework — Disorders of the Skeletal Structures — Muscles: Their Structure, Function, and Diseases — How the Body Derives Its Energy

SECTION VII—The Skin and Its Diseases

The Body's Covering — Skin Diseases

SECTION VIII—Urinary and Sex Organs

The Urinary Organs — Diseases of the Urinary Organs — The Sex Organs: Male and Female — Diseases of the Male Sex Organs — Diseases of the Female Sex Organs — Sexually Transmitted Diseases

PROMINENT ACHIEVEMENTS IN MEDICINE
(A Pictorial Supplement)

SELECTIVE ATLAS OF NORMAL ANATOMY

GENERAL INDEX

# Volume 3—More Diseases; First Aid; Emergencies

SECTION I—The Glands and the Nervous System

The Glands — Endocrine Gland Disorders — The Nervous System — Diseases of the Nervous System — Mental Illness: Neuroses and Psychoses

SECTION II—The Sensory System

The Organs of Sensation — Pain — Diseases of the Eye — Diseases of the Ear, Nose, and Throat

SECTION III—Cancer

Characteristics of Cancer — Manifestations of Cancer

SECTION IV—Dietary Problems

Deficiency Diseases — Disorders of Regulation

SECTION V—Allergies and Infections

Allergic Manifestations — Infections — Viral Diseases — Rickettsial and Chlamydial Diseases — Bacterial Diseases — Systemic Fungal Diseases — Parasitic Infections

SECTION VI—First Aid; Poisoning; Emergencies

First-Aid Kits and Home Medicine Chests — Poisonings — First Aid for Emergencies

SECTION VII—Home Treatments

When Someone in Your Home is Ill — Simple Home Treatments

HUMAN ANATOMY—"TRANS-VISION" CHARTS

ILLUSTRATED STUDY OF CELLS

GENERAL INDEX

APPENDIX: MEDICAL INFORMATION UPDATE

# The Perpetuation
# of Life

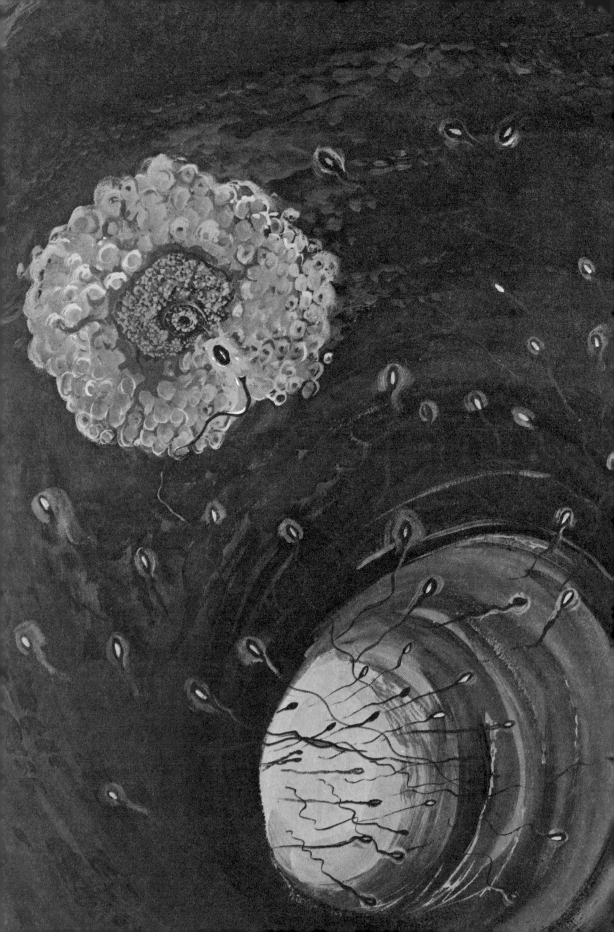

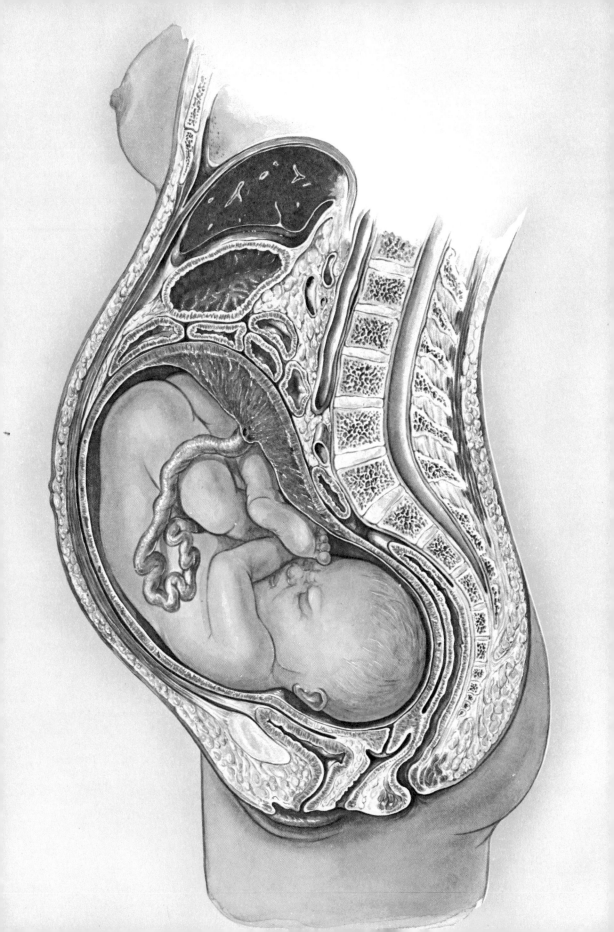

siderable loss of blood at this time. The doctor, or the nurse, often manipulates the uterus by pressure through the abdominal wall in order to make sure that it contracts firmly.

*What Is an Episiotomy?* In some cases the tissues which stretch to form the birth canal are not sufficiently elastic to accommodate the child's head. They offer resistance to the descent of the head. But with the tremendous pressure produced by the contraction of the uterine muscle, the child's head keeps on making progress in spite of this resistance. If there is no intervention, these tissues will eventually tear as they make room for the head to pass through. The physician in charge of the delivery will guard against this possibility and will usually prefer to make an incision rather than permit the tissues to tear. The making of such an incision to enlarge the birth canal is spoken of as an episiotomy.

After the third stage of labor, the incision is repaired by stitches. Thus restored, the tissues resume their normal shape and position. The area will be tender, of course, for several weeks after the delivery, but the final result is much better than if the tissues had been allowed to tear of their own accord.

*What Is a Cesarean Operation?* A cesarean operation is a procedure for delivering a baby by surgery rather than allowing it to pass through the birth canal in the usual manner. The doctor makes an incision through the abdominal wall and then through the uterus into the cavity which contains the child. The operation, a major surgical procedure, requires one of the forms of general or regional anesthesia. The child is removed through the incisions that have been made, and then the placenta and protective membranes are separated from the uterus and removed. The uterus is caused to contract to prevent bleeding, and the incisions are closed with stitches.

Physicians once considered the cesarean operation an emergency measure to be used only when childbirth by the usual route was impossible. In more recent years, techniques have been perfected until the procedure has become relatively safe. When a problem develops at the time of childbirth, the doctor must decide which is better—to allow delivery in the regular way or to intervene by surgery. Cesarean cases must stay in the hospital a little longer than others.

*The Baby's Position During Birth.* A baby may be in any one of several positions at the time of its birth. Usually and fortunately, its head passes through the birth canal first. Being firm and round, it serves more effectively to stretch the soft tissues of the mother's pelvic organs than would some other part of the infant's body. As mentioned above, the baby's head is usually in an oblique plane with respect to the mother's pelvis. Its face may be directed either forward or backward with respect to the mother. The process of birth is a little easier when the infant's face is directed backward.

In a small percentage of deliveries the child's buttocks pass through the birth canal first. Such a case is called a "breech presentation," and labor is more difficult than when the head comes first. Sometimes the doctor in charge will recommend a cesarean operation rather than permit the longer, more difficult delivery which a breech presentation involves.

In still a smaller number of cases, the child's shoulders or some other part of his body lies across the birth canal at the time labor begins. In such event, the doctor must choose between an internal manipulation of the child or the cesarean operation.

**Changes in the Child's Body**

Several major changes take place within an infant's body at the time of birth. The most striking of these involves the expansion of the lungs so that henceforth the infant obtains oxygen directly from breathing air instead of getting it by a transfer between the

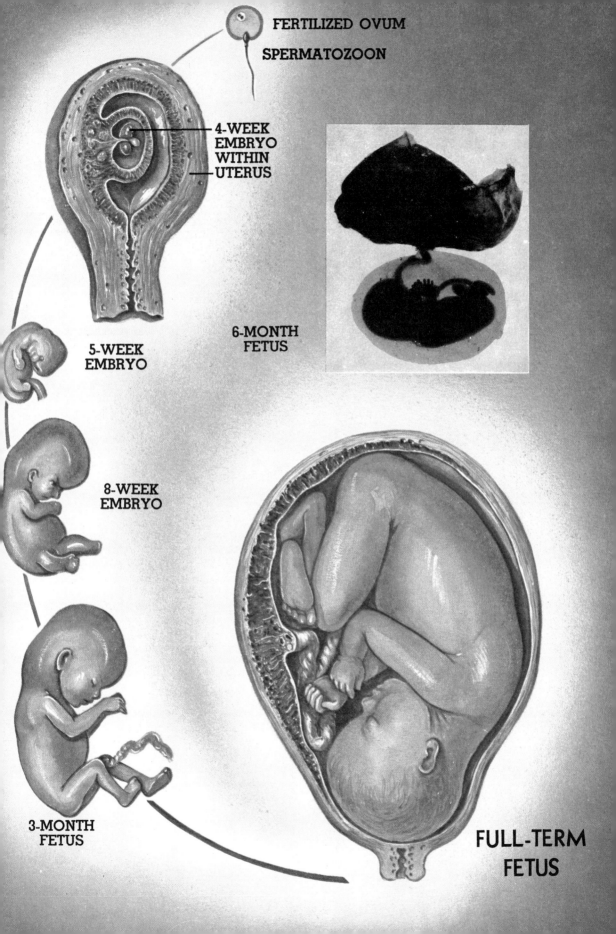

FERTILIZED OVUM

SPERMATOZOON

4-WEEK
EMBRYO
WITHIN
UTERUS

6-MONTH
FETUS

5-WEEK
EMBRYO

8-WEEK
EMBRYO

3-MONTH
FETUS

FULL-TERM
FETUS

few new structures develop during this time, for the organs and tissues of the new body have been well established during the first three months.

### The Plan of Fetal Circulation

The route which the blood follows through the body of a fetus differs markedly from that which it will follow after birth. A word about this now will prepare the way for understanding the circulatory changes that will occur at the time of birth.

In the fetus the purest blood is that

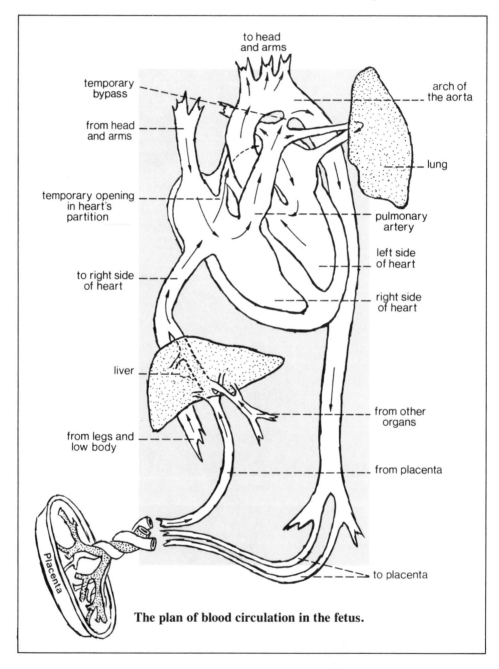

The plan of blood circulation in the fetus.

not receive the modern treatment of an injection of Rh immune globulin within 72 hours of the delivery of her first child, she will build up antibodies in her blood which will endanger the child of her next pregnancy.

In the present chapter we are concerned with the illness itself as it may affect a second or third child born to a mother who has not received the protective injection just mentioned.

There are various degrees of this illness, from mild to so severe that the child does not survive. The milder cases are typically those born in a second pregnancy, whereas the more severe cases are those born in subsequent pregnancies. The baby with a moderate to severe form of this disease is often born prematurely and, as in the case of other premature births, is especially susceptible to the respiratory distress syndrome, discussed later in this chapter under "Respiratory Problems." The baby is extremely pale, and there is generalized swelling (edema) of the tissues of his body to the extent that it is difficult for the child's elbows and knees to bend. The liver and spleen are both enlarged. Blood tests show a large amount of bilirubin in the infant's blood, this being one of the chemical by-products of the breakdown of hemoglobin which results from the destruction of red blood cells by the antibodies which the child received from its mother.

In the treatment of a child born with hemolytic disease it is important to flush out the antibodies and the high concentrations of bilirubin in the infant's blood. This cleansing is accomplished by the procedure of exchange transfusion, in which the infant's own blood is replaced. It is important that this procedure be carried out as soon as possible, for a continued high concentration of bilirubin predisposes to the serious disease of kernicterus, in which the child's brain suffers damage.

### Systemic Infections

The newborn baby is particularly susceptible to systemic infections be-cause there has not yet been time for the full development of his immune mechanisms—the body's defenses against invasion by microorganisms. The infant born prematurely is even more susceptible to infections than one born at full term. Systemic infections account for 10 to 20 percent of deaths

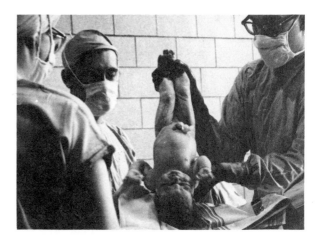

occurring in newborn babies. Even with modern methods of treatment, the mortality rate for such cases stands at about 40 percent.

Systemic infections are caused by an invasion of bacteria or viruses into the baby's tissues by any one of several routes (umbilicus, throat, eye membranes), either before birth, at the time of delivery, or within a few days after the child is born.

In the newborn baby, the symptoms of systemic infection are often vague and may include loss of appetite, restlessness, fluctuations in body temperature (with low temperature being more common than fever), vomiting, diarrhea, and difficult breathing.

Infections caused by group B streptococcus germs typically take the form of pneumonia or of meningitis. Those caused by the staphylococcus often cause a breakdown of some area of the baby's skin.

It is urgent that the infant with systemic infection be under a doctor's

# Patterns of Growth and Development

We have earlier traced, in chapter 4, the complicated plan of human development which occurs during the first three months following conception. During this period the fundamental tissues and organs are formed. The fetus then resembles a newborn child except for differing proportions in the various parts of its body.

In the present chapter we will consider the continuing phases of growth and development through the remainder of fetal life and in the periods of infancy, childhood, and adolescence. We will observe that at certain times growth takes place more rapidly than at other times. The organ systems follow their individual patterns of development, with some progressing at a faster rate than others. Also there are certain male and female differences. Even within the same sex some individuals develop at a faster rate than others.

### The Control of Growth and Development

The *basic pattern* of an individual's growth and development is determined by the combination of chromosomes and genes at the time of his conception. Whether he will be tall or stocky or of athletic build is a matter of heredity. The hormones produced by the endo-crine organs also influence a person's growth and development.

### Endocrine Influences in Growth

Beginning at about two years of age the growth hormone produced by the anterior pituitary gland and the thyroxine produced by the thyroid gland become important in regulating the child's growth. Excess of the growth hormone causes a child to become taller than he would normally be. Deficiencies in the growth hormone will cause the child to be smaller, perhaps even a dwarf in extreme cases. Giantism and dwarfism are explained in greater detail in chapter 2, volume 3.

Throughout the years of childhood, growth continues at a rather leisurely rate, in about the same pattern for boys as for girls. But when a child comes into his adolescent period, additional hormones are produced by the sex organs which not only stimulate the rate of growth but modify it differently for boys than for girls. It is at the beginning of adolescence that the pituitary gland produces a hormone known as gonadotropin, which stimulates the sex organs, either male or female, to produce androgens in the body of a boy and estrogens in the body of a girl.

Androgens are hormones produced

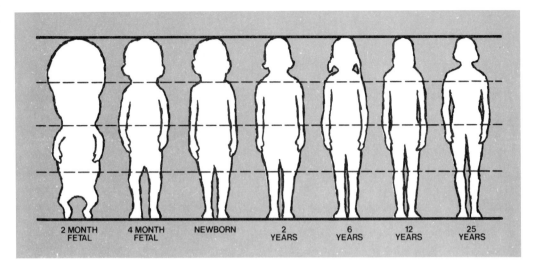

| 2 MONTH FETAL | 4 MONTH FETAL | NEWBORN | 2 YEARS | 6 YEARS | 12 YEARS | 25 YEARS |

**The proportion of head, body, and limbs changes greatly as development progresses.**

total height. The reduction does not mean, of course, that the head has decreased in size. The head has continued to grow throughout fetal life and, at a slower pace, throughout childhood. It means that the head grew faster than other parts in the early stages of development and then, growing at a slower pace, allowed the other parts to assume their share of the adult height by the time physical maturity was attained.

Significant changes take place also in the relative length of the trunk as compared with that of the limbs. During the first year after birth, it is the trunk that grows most in relative size. At one year of age, the child's large trunk and big head contrast with his short, fat legs, which are often bowed. But after this first year, the legs grow faster than other parts.

Up until the onset of adolescence, the body build of boys and girls remains similar. Of course, some are slender and some are chubby, but this variation occurs in boys as well as in girls. But beginning at adolescence, when the growth spurt occurs, the developing young male follows a different pattern from that of the developing young female.

Girls arrive at their adolescent time of life two and a half years sooner, on the average, than boys. This earlier onset of adolescence accounts for two interesting observations. First, for a short time in the early teens girls are larger and taller than boys of the same age. Second, boys, on the average, remain for a longer period than girls in that phase of growth in which the legs are growing faster than the body. So, when both boys and girls have completed their growth spurts, the average boy is taller than the average girl, the reason being that his legs are longer. The length of the body is about the same in young men as it is in young women. That is, the sitting height of an average young man is essentially the same as the sitting height of an average young woman.

Another difference in the proportions of a young man's body as compared with a young woman's is in the greater breadth of his shoulders. Because of his broader shoulders, it appears that a man has narrower hips than does a woman. Actually, the breadth of the hips is essentially the same for an average man as for an average woman.

83

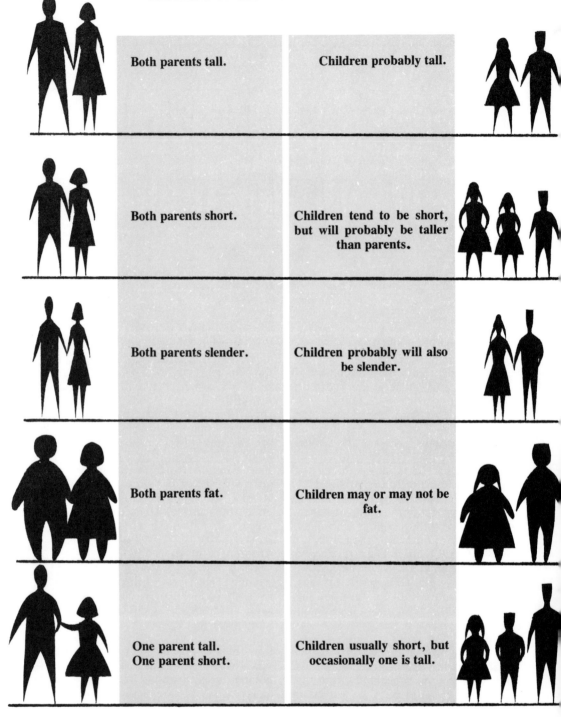

| | |
|---|---|
| Both parents tall. | Children probably tall. |
| Both parents short. | Children tend to be short, but will probably be taller than parents. |
| Both parents slender. | Children probably will also be slender. |
| Both parents fat. | Children may or may not be fat. |
| One parent tall. One parent short. | Children usually short, but occasionally one is tall. |

Many times a child inherits a tendency to be tall or short, fat or slender. The diagrams above give a hint on what to expect.

SECTION **III**

# On Being
# Good Parents

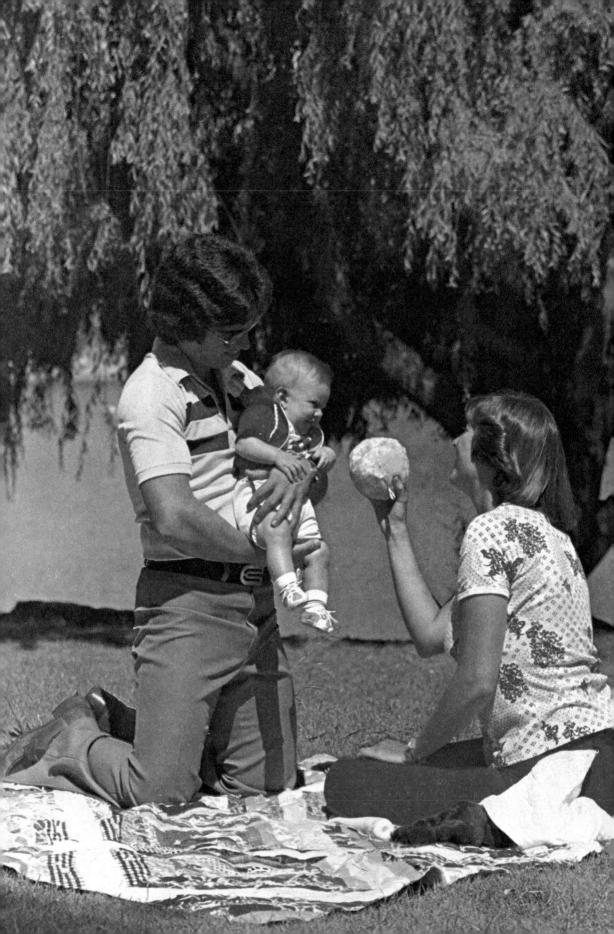

# The Philosophy of Parenthood

"Why do you want to get married?" I asked rather bluntly of a young couple who sat in my office telling about their plans for marriage.

They looked at each other as much as to ask, "How dumb can he be?"

I admit that the question was unnecessary as a means of obtaining information. But I wanted them to focus attention on certain important considerations in their immediate planning.

The desire that prompts a young man and a young woman who love each other to unite their lives in marriage comes from God. And if they will use their good judgment not only in their selection of each other for life partners but also in their plans for marriage and their conduct of a home, their personal happiness will be greatly increased by sharing life together. The Scripture says, "It is not good that the man should be alone." Genesis 3:18.

Just as sharing life together in marriage increases the happiness of a man and a woman, so sharing their life with children increases the happiness of husband and wife. The desire to be parents also comes from God.

In order to realize the increased happiness which parenthood can provide, parents must use good judgment as they establish the policies of their home

and as they deal wisely and kindly with their children.

Parenthood provides many rewards. Among these is the evidence of personal adequacy.

The early teenager, as he begins to realize that he must face life on his own, naturally asks, Am I equal to successful living? This question bothers some teenagers more than others. The bolder, self-reliant type usually dismisses the question casually with the expectation that he will make the most of his social opportunities and thus ensure for himself a place among his fellows.

The quiet, timid youth, on the contrary, may not find his way through to the answer so confidently. Even though he is doing well in school and even though he has a group of loyal friends of his own sex and age, he may harbor serious doubt about his ability to carve out a niche for himself in the stern world that he sees around him.

As young people reach their late teens, be they extrovert or introvert, their participation in social affairs begins to give them assurance that they are well received and that they are personally adequate. When a boy asks a girl for a date and she accepts, both the boy and the girl feel complimented—

# The Father's Part

*Is being a father just an honorary position? Do modern families need a father who carries his share of responsibility for directing the family's activities? Or is being "head of the house" only a figurehead job? Are not mothers, nowadays, directing the affairs of the household as effeciently as did the father-mother team of former years? Does the present-day father's job consist, essentially, of simply providing financial support for the family?* These and many similar questions could be asked to underscore the need for and value of a frank discussion of the father's part in modern family life.

In one case of grave misunderstanding on the subject, the husband accused his wife of being arbitrary in the discipline of the children. "She gives them spankings every day whether they need them or not," this father complained. "I think she is ruining their dispositions because she requires them to do this and do that and keeps them upset about half the time."

The mother countered that her husband, always busy with his professional duties, hardly ever stayed home. She said, "I want my husband to succeed in his career, but I don't think it is fair for him to criticize me when I have to carry the whole burden of the home and of the children without his help."

## The Pattern Has Changed

In the days when most Americans lived in the country, it was easy and natural for a father to spend much time with his children. Even though the typical father of seventy-five years ago worked from morning until night, his work usually kept him at home or near home, and thus the children could be with him much of the time. Probably the boys spent more time with their father because they could help him with his work. But in many rural families the girls worked out-of-doors almost as much as the boys. Anyway, families remained close-knit, and all members worked cooperatively in the struggle to make a living.

But with the coming of urbanization and automation, the father no longer earns the living at home. Now he punches a time clock or sits behind a desk in surroundings in which children would be out of place. In many families, both the father and mother leave home about the time the children wake up and arrive back home just in time to pick them up from the baby-sitter. With the money they earn the family is fed, clothed, and housed. The father is tempted to reason, What more can children ask of a father than to provide their support?

But the shift from country living to

the boy because of evidence that the girl considers him to be her social equal, and the girl because she now knows that she is admired by a boy she likes.

When the courtship leads to marriage, the fact of marriage provides for young people the best possible answer to all their previous questions about adequacy and acceptance by others. With confidence resting on a completed romance, they feel ready to face whatever the world demands.

Many a young man who otherwise would have become discouraged has pressed on to final success because of the encouragement of his loyal wife. Similarly, a young wife expresses her appreciation of her husband by becoming the best homemaker possible.

Then comes parenthood! Just as marriage provides real evidence that a young man and a young woman are socially acceptable, so the coming of the first child provides reassurance that the two members of this partnership are biologically adequate. The spontaneous love for the child which fills the heart of both the young father and the young mother as they hold their first-born in their arms is a composite of many deep-rooted feelings. It includes gratitude for God's care over the young mother's life during the experience of childbirth. It includes their happiness in the fulfillment of their plans for parenthood. And it includes their feelings of personal reassurance now that they have been privileged to pass on the spark of life to the first member of the next generation in their own home.

### Parents Appreciate Each Other More

A newly married husband and wife tend, still, to identify with the families from which they came. When a young wife speaks of "my family," she refers to the home of her childhood. But once this same young woman becomes a mother she speaks differently. It is now "our family" and "we three."

A husband and wife, of course, never become blood relatives. They are not related to each other in the sense that

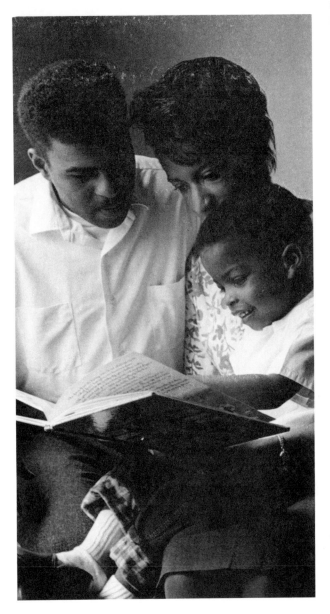

they have the same grandfather or the same Aunt Jane. But the coming of the first child unites their lives in an even more intimate relationship than that of blood relatives. Now they are most definitely related because they are mother and father to the same child. Furthermore, they have achieved parenthood not by individual ability but as a united undertaking.

94

# *Discussing Intimate Matters*

Four-year-old Tommy looked up from his play and asked his mother, "Did you know before I was born that I was going to be a boy?"

It happened that a neighbor lady with a new baby had been visiting earlier that day, and Tommy had overheard the conversation. The two mothers had mentioned that the new baby was the first girl in a family with three boys.

"No, I didn't know before you were born whether you were a girl or a boy," Tommy's mother admitted. "But I am glad you are a boy," she continued, "just as glad over your being a boy as I am that your sister is a girl."

Here was a wise mother who gave her child a simple, honest answer. Such an answer would probably satisfy the curiosity of any Tommy for several days or weeks. But eventually the child will ask more questions along these lines. When he does, the mother should reply in a similar, matter-of-fact way.

## Childhood Curiosity

Children are normally and naturally curious about the origin of life as well as about the parts of their bodies that make boys different from girls.

Many parents feel inadequate when asked to explain the biological facts of life. It is unfortunate, however, for a parent to disappoint his child by giving vague answers. The curiosity which prompts the questions is strong, and if parents miss such natural opportunities to guide the child's understanding, the child will take his questions to someone else. Or later on the parents may have to face the awkwardness of a contrived session to discuss these intimate matters.

Some parents think that the facts of life are an improper topic for discussion. But the human body is God's handiwork of creation, and it is proper that a child should learn about it and how it operates. It is best that he learn from his parents rather than from persons whose ideals and information are questionable.

When a parent throws an air of mystery around conversations on life and sex, or taboos them, the child is placed at a disadvantage. Many a young woman has found adjustment to her own marriage difficult because, when she was a girl, the mother implanted the idea that sex is vulgar. A young man may be tempted to "sow his wild oats" for no other reason than that his father failed to satisfy his boyhood questions about sex. Here, even more than in other phases of life, parents have a definite molding influence on their children. And this influence is exerted as much as by example and attitude as by words. In the home where the father and mother are congenial and express their affection for each other and for the children in casual, natural ways, the children will develop wholesome attitudes toward marriage and sex.

### When to Begin Sex Education

Sex education in the broad sense consists of preparing a child to live comfortably with other people of both sexes, to be a sensible lover when he reaches the age of romance, and eventually to be a good husband or wife. Sex education really begins on the first day of a child's life. An infant should be loved, fondled, held close, and made to feel that he belongs. Even when he cannot use language to express and receive ideas, the foundations of his personality and of his future ability to be at ease with people are being laid.

Sex instruction has a physical component as well as an emotional one. The parents' attitude as they meet the infant's physical needs has a subtle influence on the budding personality. When the mother manifests disgust at changing the diapers and when she hurries through feeding times as though she had something more important to do, she unknowingly contributes to an attitude in which the child thinks of his body as being repulsive.

A mother should be casual as she handles the infant or young child at bath time. She should not draw undue attention to the sensitive parts of his body, and she should try to make the experience a comfortable one in which the child feels at ease even when his entire body is exposed.

It is quite natural for an infant, as he becomes aware of his surroundings, to explore the various parts of his body. There even comes a time when he seems to pay undue attention to his genital areas. It is easy for a parent at such a time, to become alarmed, to express disgust, and to chastise the child

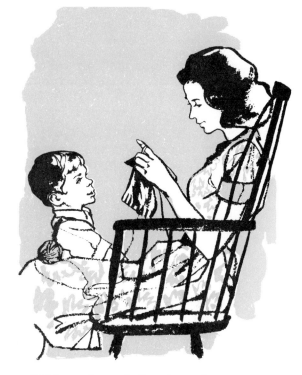

"Did you know before I was born that I was going to be a boy?"

as though he had committed some wrong. At this early stage, the child is innocent in such a matter and being reprimanded only tends to focus his attention and encourage his curiosity. Thus it will be easy for him to experiment secretly as he tries to find the reason why his parent scolded him earlier.

The wise parent will show no surprise as the young child explores the parts of his body and will tactfully draw his interest to something else rather than allow him time to overindulge his curiosity.

As a child begins to talk, he learns words that pertain to the intimate parts of his body and to the functions of elimination. Some parents use babytalk words for this part of the child's vocabulary. It is easy for such words to persist until a child reaches school age, and then he becomes embarrassed for

"How does a baby start?" is a question most parents think requires a brief course in biology. Actually, however, the child may not benefit too much by a long answer about the birds and bees. The child wants a direct answer and a reasonably simple one. When the child already knows that the unborn baby develops within the body of its mother, he can now be told that the new baby starts from a cell something like a seed. It can be explained that this seed has two parts, one from the mother and one from the father. These two parts join inside the mother's body and the cell begins to grow and make other cells, until pretty soon there are enough cells to make a tiny baby. This much of an explanation will usually satisfy for a while, but eventually there will be other questions.

The question which parents seem to dread most is, "How does the father's part of the seed get into the mother?" The answer should be as simple as possible.

The parent can say, "You know how a boy's body is made and you know that it is different from a girl's body. The bodies of a husband and wife are like the bodies of a boy and a girl. The Creator has made them in such a way that they fit together, and this allows the father's part of the seed to pass into the mother's body, where it joins the mother's part of the seed."

Some children are particularly curious about the process of birth. The diagrams in chapters 4 and 5 of this volume will be helpful in answering the child's questions on how the baby gets out of the mothers's body.

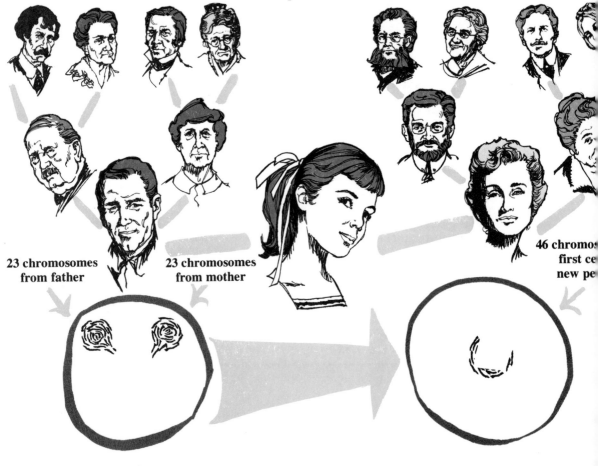

When the sex cells of a father and a mother unite to form a new life, they make it possible for the child to inherit traits from each parent and each parent's ancestors.

23 chromosomes from father

23 chromosomes from mother

46 chromos͟ first ce͟ new pe͟

ture rather than the positive, wholesome side. It calls for a lot of tact and good common sense.

## Parents Set the Pace

The attitudes maintained at home, including off-the-record remarks by parents, go far to establish a child's patterns of future conduct. When a father and mother respect each other and manifest the type of love in the home which is both pure and filled with appreciation, the children growing up in that home will adopt for themselves similar attitudes and standards of behavior.

But if parents, even with innocent motives, permit themselves to use the facts of life as the basis for joking, or if in casual conversation they cast reflection on marriage, the child may accept this example as an excuse for having his own questionable standards for intimate matters.

# Preparing the Child for Life

Gradually, during the early months and years of a child's life, mental and physical powers develop. Soon the child becomes able to think clearly, to express himself, and to have opinions of his own. But even yet he does not have good judgment. This attribute comes by experience, a commodity still in short supply because the child has not yet lived long enough. The parents, one generation ahead of the child, have had the experience necessary to help the child develop his understanding of the meaning of life. They should, therefore, transfer the benefits of this greater experience to the child, patiently coaching him in the making of wise choices. With good guidance a child becomes more able, year by year, to carry responsibility for his own activities. By the time he reaches his late teens and early twenties he should be prepared to act wisely in making life's major decisions: the choice of a lifework, the choice of a life companion, and (most important of all) the choice of his personal philosophy.

Educators and sociologists generally recognize that of the many factors influencing a child during the period of his development, the influence of the home stands out above even that of the church or the school. Communities consist of individual homes. And only as homes establish and maintain high ideals will the nation remain strong enough to withstand the influences of greed and lawlessness.

## Caution Against Two Extremes

Parents need to avoid two extremes as they develop the policies of their home. One is that of sidestepping the responsibilities of parenthood by allowing the child to grow up as he pleases. Permissiveness, we call it.

The opposite extreme, which wise parents will also avoid, is that of rigidly controlling each detail of a child's conduct right through the years of adolescence. Parents who adopt this extreme mistakenly believe that the goal in child training is to make their children comply with their own concepts of perfect behavior. Such parents expect their children to make no mistakes. They make no allowance for a child's personal preferences.

Instead of conforming to either of these extremes in child training, parents should choose a broad and far-reaching course. Their duty is to prepare their children for successful living—not to force them to comply, puppet fashion, to an arbitrary list of dos and don'ts, nor to allow them to grow up with little or no restraint at all.

### A Child's Developing Conscience

A child's conscience is not handed to him ready-made. Conscience is that element in personality that prompts an individual to act in harmony with what he believes to be right. In order to have a trustworthy conscience then, a person must first develop the ideals on which his code of conduct is based.

Once developed, conscience enables a person to measure his choices and activities by comparison with his personal code. If a certain proposal is consistent with one's established pattern, conscience at once approves. Thus it might even approve of telling a lie to

**Erasing the barrier between the two generations reduces the problems of discipline.**

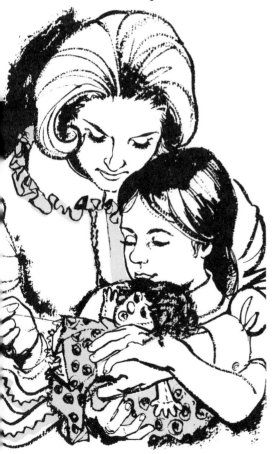

save face, if one's personal code did not forbid. But, on the other hand, if conscience has been trained against lying, it would dictate a decision in favor of telling the truth rather than distorting it, even at the expense of some humiliation or loss.

A young child's conscience, therefore, has to be developed. This presents parents with an opportunity, as well as an awesome responsibility, to help their child understand what is acceptable and what is not. Their early training establishes in the child the first vestiges of conscience by which he classes certain things as "right" and others as "wrong."

Throughout the formative years of a child's life, the parent has opportunity to help the child round out his personal code. Then as the child becomes old enough to assume responsibility for his own way of life, he will have to decide whether or not the code which his parents helped him to form is the one he will follow the rest of his life.

Whether or not a child is satisfied with this code will depend in large part on his appraisal of his parents as individuals. If, in his opinion, they represent the kind of person he wants to be, then he will accept their code of ethics. If he feels dissatisfied with his parents' way of life, then he will change the code which they have taught him. In any event, the influence of the parents' early training will stay with a child, in one way or another, throughout life. The basic framework of character around which a child builds his pattern of life has been established.

As parents help to guide a child in his understanding of what is "right" and what is "wrong," they are naturally influenced by their own religious beliefs. It is perfectly proper for parents to present their beliefs to their children in as convincing a manner as possible. Teaching a child to be religious gives him the greatest stabilizing influence of his life. True, the child, as he comes to maturity, may not choose to follow his parents' religion. But if his parents have been consistent in practicing their

# Hazards of Homelife

Each year in the United States approximately 100,000 deaths result from accidents of all kinds. For persons between the ages of 1 and 44, accidents rate as the most common cause of death. For persons of all ages, accidents stand in fourth place as a cause of death, being exceeded only by heart disease, cancer, and stroke.

Traditionally home is a quiet, peaceful, and safe place to be. Parents and children spend a great deal of time there. Tragically, however, an estimated 21 million Americans are involved each year in accidents that occur at home. Of these, about 25,000 die and about 100,000 are disabled. Home accidents are the second most common cause of accidental death, motor-vehicle accidents being the first.

Great safety campaigns pioneered and sponsored by industry have proved that accidents can be prevented, at least among industrial employees. This knowledge should encourage parents also to carry on safety campaigns in their homes and thus bring about a similar reduction in the number of domestic accidents. It is significant that adults (including parents) are involved in a great many of the accidents at home. Thus, parents should first take the matter to heart and then teach their children by example as well as by precept.

We tend to judge the dangers that threaten life and health by comparing the number of fatalities from one cause with those from another. But in doing so we forget that, particularly in the case of accidents, there are many times more injuries than deaths. And these injuries, even though not fatal, cause suffering, loss of time from school or employment, and often permanent handicaps.

Before we launch into a consideration of the individual hazards of homelife, let us mention the types of accidental death that affect the various age groups.

For infants under one year of age, the accident rate, though high, is overshadowed by other causes of death. Nevertheless, accidents do take their toll here also, two types being especially threatening: (1) suffocation by bedclothes, pillows, and from being lain on; (2) injury from objects that have been swallowed. These two categories taken together account for about two thirds of all accidental deaths for children under one year of age.

In the one- to four-year-old group, motor vehicle accidents constitute the principal cause of death. Though most of these do not occur at home, still a fair percentage do—in the driveway or at the curb as the child is run over by a car. Burns, scalds, and drownings are also important causes of accidental death at this age. In the five- to four-teen-year-old group, motor vehicle mishaps still account for the greatest number of accidental deaths. Drownings come second, with firearm accidents and burns in third and fourth place.

For youth from fifteen to twenty-four years of age, motor vehicle accidents and drownings still hold first and sec-ond places. Firearms accidents and falls take a considerable toll as well.

For adults, falls cause the greatest number of domestic accidental deaths. Fire comes second, and death from suf-focation or strangulation, third. The fourth most common cause of fatal home accidents for women is poison-ing; for men, firearm accidents. Death from accidental gas poisoning comes fifth.

### Poisonings

Most accidental poisonings occur at home. The number of such cases has become so large that some authorities speak of the problem as ''an epi-demic.'' Fortunately, most cases do not end in death, but an estimated one million persons each year in the United States become poisoned in one way or another.

Poisoning by medicines kept around the house occurs most commonly in young children. Toddlers under three have a natural urge to put things in their mouths. They may have seen their parents help themselves to the contents of a medicine bottle, and they feel that they can do likewise. In older children and adults the hazard of unlabeled bot-tles accounts for many cases of poison-ing. For children, the common aspirin bottle provides the greatest temptation and danger. Even though aspirin is sup-posed to be relatively harmless, yet several tablets taken at a time can easily cause fatal poisoning.

Other agents around the house be-sides medicines that cause poisoning are the bright-color pigments used in

## RULES FOR SAFE SWIMMING

1. Have a medical examination before you learn to swim.

2. Do not swim alone and do not swim when you are tired, overheated, or chilled.

3. Do not jump or dive into water that may be so cold that it will numb your body. Instead, ease into the water gradually. Do not swim long distances in cold water—it is too exhausting.

4. If you get very tired, try floating for a few minutes or at least change your style of swimming.

5. If your leg muscles cramp, draw your knees up toward your chest. Massage and move your cramped leg while you are in ''face float'' position.

6. Do not dive into water that is less than eight feet deep.

7. Never dive into water where there may be hidden rocks or logs.

8. Avoid swimming in the dark.

9. Do not joke by calling for help. Save this call for the time when you may actually need help.

# POISONINGS

See Chapter 22 of

Volume 3

for

First Aid

Symptoms

Treatment

OF POISONINGS

coloring decorations and ornaments, and the fluid contained in bubbling Christmas-tree lights. Also hair sprays, underarm sprays, insect repellents, cleaning solvents, kerosene, and bleaches are poisonous when taken into the body. Improperly vented fuel-burning heaters, regardless of what fuel is used, can give off poisonous carbon monoxide gas. The same gas from a car motor thoughtlessly left running inside a garage can have lethal effects, even in the house if the garage is connected to it.

The symptoms and treatments of the common poisonous agents are discussed in volume 3, chapter 22. But even though many lives can be saved by prompt action after a poison has been taken into the body, the ideal means of preventing illness and death from this cause is for parents to place beyond a child's reach all medicines and other toxic agents.

**Three safe ways to help a swimmer in distress.**

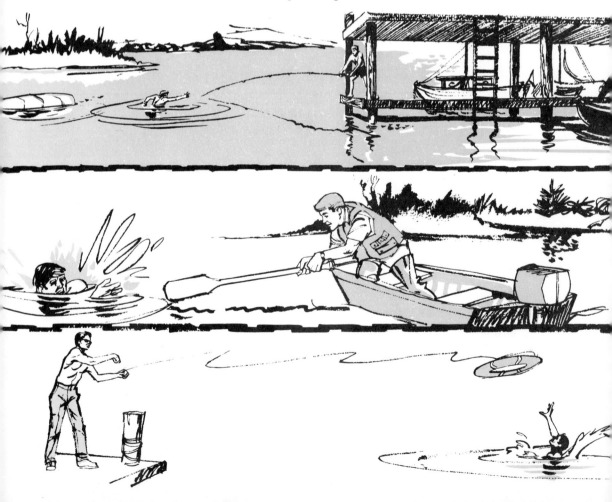

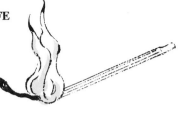

## Fire and Burns

Prevention is the best way to combat the hazard of fire in the home. Any successful program must start with instruction in fire safety and depends upon the attitude, willingness, and energy of the parents. The following points should be included in any program of instruction:

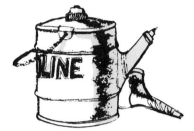

A. DANGERS. Many conditions and circumstances may prevail in a home making it vulnerable to fire. The most important of these can be listed as follows:

1. *The careless use of cigarettes and matches.* In most fires caused by the mishandling of matches, the guilty parties were under five years of age. Fires caused by cigarettes often start in the bedroom when a person smokes after retiring. Many flammable materials brought in contact with a burning cigarette ignite like kindling.

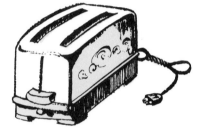

2. *Piles of rubbish or discarded items in the attic, in the basement, or in any other part of the house or garage.* One of the most effective steps in fire prevention is to keep the house and garage tidy.

3. *Oily rags, particularly those used in painting, or any materials soaked with the drying oils used in painting.* These may catch fire by spontaneous combustion even though no spark is present. Promptly after use such materials should be discarded in a fireproof container or destroyed by burning.

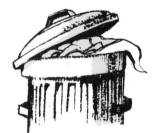

4. *Heating equipment in poor repair.* This danger may involve a faulty

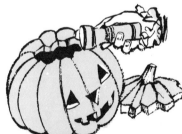

**Matches are dangerous.**

**Never start fires with gasoline or kerosene.**

**Electrical equipment should be repaired by an electrician.**

**Keep covered. Put oily rags in metal cans.**

**Halloween masks and costumes burn easily—use a flashlight.**

**Use a screen to protect a fireplace.**

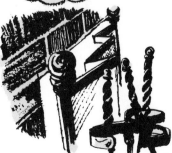

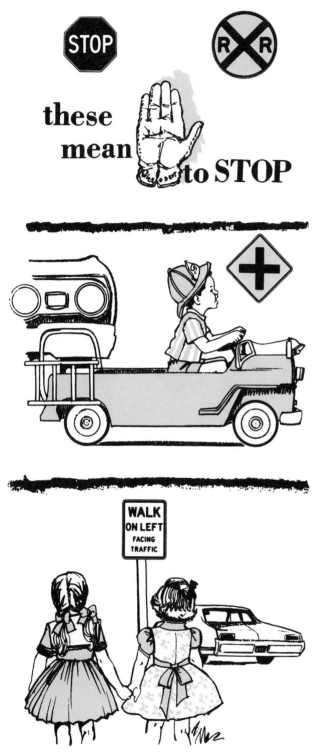

**Safety rules must be taught early.**

have the fatal driveway accidents in which an adult moves the car without realizing a child is in the driver's blind spot. Also, we have here the tragedies in which a child runs between parked cars into the path of a moving vehicle. Parental precautions, admonitions, and watchcare could reduce these accidents materially.

If your young school-age child walks between home and school, it would be well for you to walk with him at the beginning of each new school session and occasionally thereafter to make sure that he is following the safest route and that he understands where and how to protect himself from the dangers of moving traffic.

If he rides to and from school, he faces the greatest danger when entering and leaving the vehicle. He should be instructed to enter and leave only on the curb side and not to move around the vehicle, if this ever becomes necessary, until perfectly sure no car is coming.

The number of bicycles in the United States has increased enormously in recent years. The bicyclist is at a disadvantage when riding with other vehicles on city streets or country highways. Therefore it is not surprising that in any one year about one out of ten cyclists will meet with some mishap serious enough to require professional medical treatment.

Many fatal bicycle accidents result from collision with automobiles. Others are caused by double riding, improper braking, stunting, faulty mechanical condition of the bicycle, or by the rider's losing control or becoming entangled in moving parts of the bicycle.

A parent's effort is well spent in training the child who rides a bicycle to follow the traffic rules intended for motorists—riding on the right side of the street, obeying traffic signals, and using arm signals before making a turn.

Fundamentally irresponsible and still lacking the balanced judgment necessary to plan their movements wisely, children are vulnerable to accidents in traffic. The parent's effort must be directed toward educating the child regarding traffic dangers and toward enforcing reasonable traffic cautions until these become automatic in the pattern of the child's behavior.

### Playtime Accidents

Danger of accidents during play will vary, of course, from one age group to another and from one type of play activity to another. Play activities at school are under the direction of the person in charge. The parents' chief responsibility, therefore, is limited to exerting an influence through the home and school organization and to encouraging and upholding the teachers and athletic supervisors in planning programs considered relatively safe.

To prevent possible accidents on a picnic, an outing, or a hike, the parents' responsibility consists of making sure that the child is properly supervised by a trustworthy adult, cautious by nature and firm in dealing with children.

Accidents most likely to occur when children are under the supervision of their parents are drownings, boating accidents, and skiing accidents. With respect to drownings, these accidents occur at all ages but particularly among teenage boys.

### Falls

Persons of all ages are subject to falls, but falls are most disastrous to an older person. Children frequently suffer broken bones when they fall, but their bones heal more readily than do those of elderly people. Falls involving head injuries may end fatally, of course, even in the younger age groups.

One study on falls indicates that about one third of such accidents occurring at home take place on the stairs or steps. Slipping on slick floors accounts for another high percentage of falls, as also does stumbling over toys or other objects left out of place. Other falls occur while using ladders in yard work or for home repairs. Cold weather

# RULES TO HELP YOU RIDE YOUR BICYCLE SAFELY

1. Keep your bicycle in good repair.
2. Wear light-colored clothing when you ride so that motorists can see you easily.
3. Use trouser clips or a chain guard to keep your slacks or trousers from catching in the moving parts of your bicycle.
4. Ride in the same direction the traffic is moving. This rule is just opposite to the one for pedestrians.
5. Obey traffic laws and signals—especially stop signs.
6. Give hand signals when turning.
7. Stay as near as possible to the curb or edge of the road.
8. Lead your bicycle across a dangerous intersection or a railroad crossing.
9. Do not ride others with you on your bicycle.
10. Never hold on to another moving vehicle or have your bicycle towed by another vehicle.
11. When you are riding with other bicyclists, ride single file.
12. Avoid bicycle stunts unless you are in a field or yard, away from all other traffic.
13. Watch out for your own safety while you are riding; do not depend on the drivers of other vehicles to watch out for you.
14. For riding at night, use lights and reflectors.
15. Park your bicycle safely so that people will not stumble over it.

# Educational and Vocational Guidance

As young parents look into the face of their newborn baby, their imaginations are fired and they picture this same child thirty-five years later, then a grown man, beloved of his wife and children, respected in the community, and acknowledged as successful among his associates. But many things have to happen in this infant's life before his parents' fond dreams can come true.

The babe, now only seven pounds and twenty inches, will be, thirty-five years later, a well-proportioned man six feet tall and about 180 pounds in weight. We say physical development is marvelous, and truly it is!

But still more remarkable is the development of a child's intellect. Here the parents, and later the child himself, play a big part in determining the outcome, either negative or positive .

In too many cases, unfortunately, intellectual development, like the physical, is allowed to take place automatically, without guidance or plan. When this happens, the end result is like the present a six-year-old boy once made for his mother. Hearing pounding and sawing, she went to see what was happening.

"I'm making something for you," the boy announced.

"But what?" she asked.

"I don't know yet," he admitted, "but it's going to be something nice."

### Early Factors in Guidance

It is important for a child to place a high value on intellectual activities. When he observes his parents reading and keeping themselves informed, he, too, may become interested in expanding his fund of knowledge. When parents choose for their heroes persons who have reached high intellectual levels, their child may develop the impression that such attainments are worthwhile.

Even the stories parents tell their children give them a clue as to what they consider important. If a story about the child's uncle places more emphasis on his childhood pranks than on his progress in school, the child reasons that school is not important in his parents' estimation. The same applies to stories read out of a book. When the heroes are persons who have developed their brains, the child may be motivated to do the same.

### Built-in Interests Should Be Encouraged

Some children surprise their parents by announcing early in life what they plan to do when they grow up. We are

SECTION V

# The Teenager

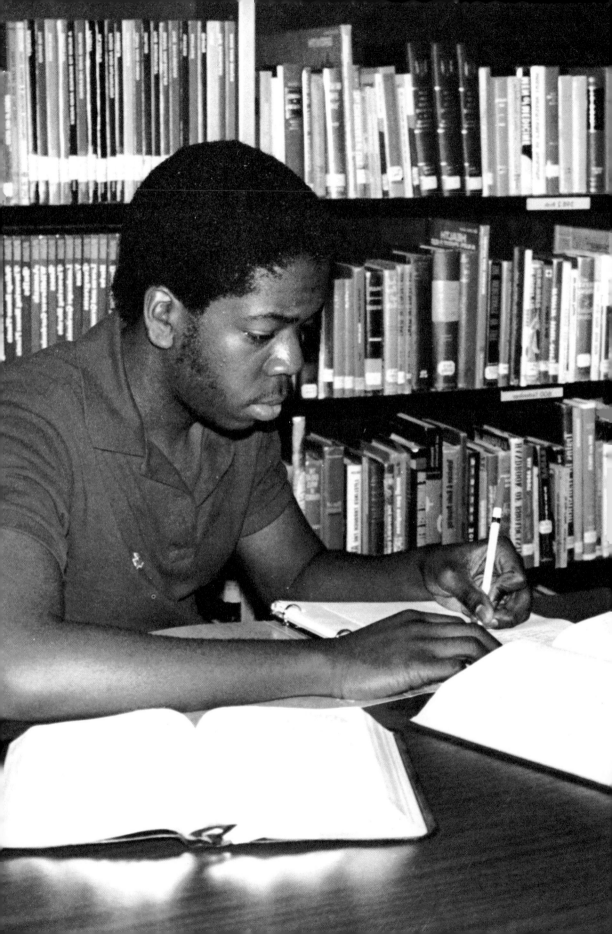

# The Urge to Experiment

A teenage boy or girl is entrusted with a new life, with its important years still in the future. If he takes good care of this valuable possession, his life will be productive and happy. If, however, through carelessness, he mars his life during this early period, he will carry a handicap throughout his remaining years.

A teenager is naturally optimistic, and to him all of life, present and future, looks rosy. He craves activity and has abundant energy. He desires to be doing things. This natural vivacity explains his urge to experiment. He is short on experience and long on curiosity. Whatever offers an opportunity to do something unusual becomes a challenge.

Not having established himself yet as a mature person, the teenager desires recognition. So he devises ways to attract attention, hoping to draw notice of one kind or another.

## What Has Happened?

Before adolescence you perhaps argued with other children about which were superior—boys or girls. Of course boys argued in favor of being boys. They considered girls to be silly. Girls gave reasons to bolster their preference for being girls, disdaining boys as thoughtless and rough.

Now that you have reached your teens, things have changed. The physical development of a girl when she reaches her early teens makes her a woman. And boys become men, though their "growing up" occurs on the average about two years later than with girls. The difference between a teenage girl and a teenage boy now shows up as much more pronounced than that between a nine-year-old girl and nine-year-old boy.

This difference between teenage boys and girls is just as marked in their personality as in their organs and physique. Interests are different; reactions are different. Upon coming into manhood or womanhood you have been mildly sensitive about the evidences that now make you a young adult. Yet you have been inwardly proud of these evidences, although at times you felt timid about laying aside the role of a child.

Now that you are in your teens, you are beginning to overcome your timidity and the attitude of rivalry. You feel a developing interest in becoming better acquainted, boys with girls and girls with boys.

It is not that a teenager is different from other human beings, but rather that his perspectives are changing, and certain qualities are coming into sharp focus. Next, therefore, we will consider the personal characteristics of the teenager.

### Curiosity

Why does a teenage boy work out on the parallel bars and practice push-ups? He has learned that the power of muscles is increased by exercise, and he desires to build up his muscles so that he can satisfy his curiosity on how strong he really can be. He knows that strength is a symbol of manhood, and he aspires to demonstrate strength equal to that of adult men.

Why does a teenage girl spend so many hours before the mirror? Because she, too, is curious over the way she will be received by others now that she is coming into the prime of womanhood with its accompanying beauty and feminine attractiveness.

Curiosity has its influence on a teenager's pattern of life. He realizes that he is short on experience, and for this reason he wants to experiment—so that he can add new experiences to what has happened already in his life. Thus he can broaden his knowledge of the world around him and of the ways adults do things. But experience for experience's sake can easily get a teenager into difficulty. He should therefore choose his experiences with discretion.

A teenager's curiosity may prompt him to try things his parents do not approve. Curiosity may cause him to experiment with drugs. It may prompt him to tamper with sex, or to read the kind of books and magazines that undermine his morals and acquaint him with vice.

In the matter of habit formation, there always has to be a first time. The helplessness of the alcoholic could never have developed had it not been for that first drink. The smoker who now realizes that smoking is damaging his health and shortening his life can trace his predicament back to that first draw on a cigarette.

Curiosity itself is a desirable trait. It has a powerful influence on the way a

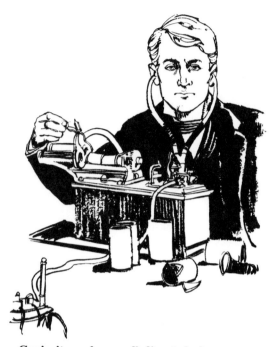

Curiosity, when well-directed, is a desirable trait. It caused Thomas Edison to become an inventor.

teenager acts. But curiosity must be balanced by sane judgment. It was while still a teenager that Thomas Edison, driven by curiosity, developed the love for science which made him a great inventor. It is curiosity over her personal capacity to please people that may prepare a teenage girl to become a charming hostess and a beloved wife and mother.

### Teenagers Are Easily Discouraged

Even with your newfound interests and your developing abilities, you may soon find that the world does not stand aside for you as much as you wish it would. Sometimes you will be brought up short with the realization that you still make mistakes. At school, there will be times when you get low marks. If you are a girl, you may find that your wonderful idea for a party is not well received by the other girls. In spite of your desire to be beautiful, you may find that you have pimples on your

nal examination until it is too late to make satisfactory preparation.

### Teenagers Crave Activity

"Why do you always want to be going places? Why can't you enjoy staying home as the rest of us like to do?" So spoke a mother to her teenage daughter who seemed always to be restless.

It is natural and normal for teenagers to seek new outlets for their energy. They need to have a variety of activities. But you must realize that this zest for activity needs to be balanced by good judgment.

Activity, of itself, can be either good or bad. So, as you give thought to becoming the kind of person you want to be, make sure that you channel your energies into activities that represent progress toward your goals. It will help you to write down a list of the things you like to do. Make the list as long as possible. Then study what you have written and make a second list placing the most important things at the top, less important things lower down, and least important at the bottom. Then, as you plan your activities, start with the things at the top of the list. You will find before you get to the bottom that you don't have time to do the less important things. This will keep you from wasting time and from neglecting the things really important to you.

### Teenagers Want Recognition

It is normal for a teenager to become impatient with restrictions. He sometimes becomes irritated with those who stand between him and his doing the things he wants to do. His desire for recognition may even bring him into difficulty. So he should be careful to earn his recognition by proper means— not by demanding it or by being a nuisance.

The teenage girl who uses gaudy makeup is using a questionable, short-cut way to attract attention and gain recognition. The wearing of "loud" clothes, use of shocking speech, free spending of pocket money, reckless

**As diners at a cafeteria must choose a balanced menu, so teenagers must choose balanced and wholesome activities.**

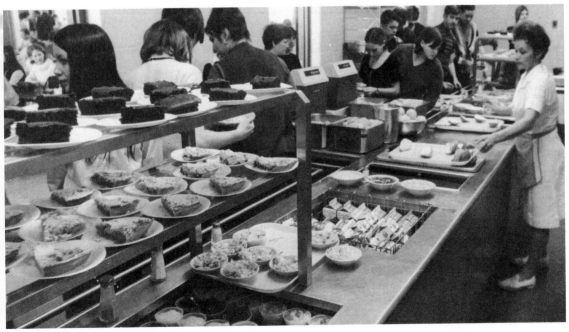

# *Petting, Pregnancy Too Soon, Homosexuality*

In this chapter we deal with the important subject of the dangers of a premature awakening of the sex responses. The related subject of masturbation has been considered in chapter 19. In the present chapter we are concerned with petting, pregnancy out of wedlock, and homosexuality. In petting, the sexual desires are stimulated by a companion of the other sex, whereas in homosexuality these desires are stimulated by one of the same sex.

## Petting

What is petting? It is variously defined by various people. For the present purpose it is defined as conduct between a man and a woman (boy and girl), in the setting of a love relationship, in which there is embracing, caressing, and fondling of the breasts or other sensitive parts of the body of one or both participants to the degree and with the result that sexual desire is aroused. Thus defined, petting does not include the act of sexual intercourse; but the aroused desire may lead to sexual intercourse if the petting is continued.

A young person should be on guard, in his personal relations with friends, against the influence of a companion who may be experienced in matters of intimate conduct. Such a person usually poses as a sincere friend. Once confidence is established, he or she uses love as an excuse for stepping over the boundary into improper conduct. In doing so, the persuasion is used, "our love for each other is so great that we must be excused for finding ways of expressing it. God gave us the capacity to love, and so no real harm can come from expressing our love to each other."

With this sort of false reassurance, an innocent young person may be easily carried along, a step at a time, until stimulation of sexual desire leads into a trap of immoral conduct without his or her realizing how it happened. Even two high-principled youths, neither of whom would think of doing anything immoral, may fall into this trap, not realizing the great strength of their sexual instincts.

It is normal and natural for a boy and a girl who admire each other to have little secrets, "just between the two of us." These may consist of a little joke, a memory of some pleasant experience, or the recalling of some embarrassing circumstance. As the friendship continues, the "secrets" may include a symbol, known only to the two of them, which stands for some expression of

The reason for mentioning this matter of venereal infection in the present instance is that teenagers, should they indulge in sexual intercourse during courtship, have not had the kind of examination by a physician that determines whether their sex organs are healthy. Many thousands of cases of venereal disease develop each year among teenagers because they have indulged in sexual intercourse not knowing that one partner or the other is infected with a venereal disease.

*Pregnancy.* Perhaps the major risk when unmarried teenagers indulge in sex is that the girl may become pregnant. Reliable estimates place the number of teenage pregnancies per year in the United States at one million, with 80 percent of them out of wedlock. This statistic gives evidence that the pregnancy in most cases was unexpected and unwanted—that it came as a surprise to the girl who indulged in sex. True, a young woman does not become pregnant every time she indulges in sex. But the point is that she does not know in advance on which occasion of sexual intercourse she will become pregnant.

By far the majority of teenagers do not welcome the prospect of parenthood. They do not indulge in sex for the sake of becoming parents. Instead, those who engage in sexual intercourse are merely experimenting with forbidden thrills. They have little or no thought at the time of the lovemaking that the result may be a pregnancy.

In a few recorded cases pregnancy has developed in girls as young as ten and eleven years of age. No group of teenagers are exempt from the possibility of pregnancy, except as they abstain from the intimacies that make pregnancy possible. Unwanted pregnancy occurs among those of every race, every creed, and every color. It occurs among those who dwell in the inner city and among those who dwell in the suburbs. It occurs among those who come from "good homes" as well as from "poor homes."

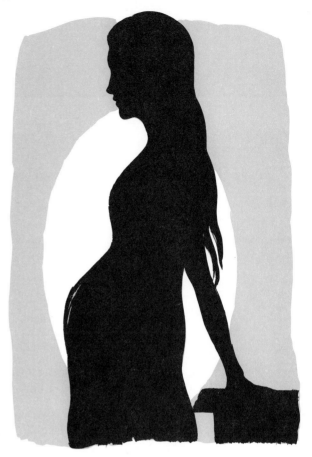

### Pregnancy out of Wedlock

Unfortunately the problems of unwanted pregnancy complicate life more for the girl than for the boy. The counsel which now follows is therefore directed quite largely to the teenage girl who becomes pregnant.

We first deal with the question, How can a girl know whether she is pregnant? Of course she will not be pregnant unless she has actually engaged in sexual intercourse. In chapter 3, page 30, this volume, we considered the early evidence of pregnancy—a missed menstrual period, a feeling of nausea and possible vomiting, and tenderness in the breasts.

A girl suspecting possible pregnancy should not wait long for these signs to develop. Her first move should be to

# Teens' Health, Health Problems, and Hazards

Teenagers should have good health. Their bodies are young. With a few exceptions, they do not carry with them, as yet, the effects of previous illnesses. But the fact remains that many of them suffer from reduced health and diminished energy.

Why should so many teenagers perform below par? For two reasons: First, the very transition from childhood to adulthood has imposed a drain on the teenager's store of vital energy. The boy who has grown fast during recent months often complains of being tired. He sometimes has headaches. He may experience pains in his joints and over his heart. The teenage girl, having recently entered womanhood, has been under more strain, both physically and nervously, than she may realize. The onset of menstruation, with loss of blood each month, may have caused her to become anemic. Stressful concern over whether she is normal, whether she will become an attractive young woman, whether she will grow too tall or too fat has wasted vital energy.

The second reason: Teenagers often tend to be careless about taking care of their bodies. Most of them follow a way of life that does more to break down their health than to promote it. Having just come into young adulthood, they don't like to acknowledge their personal limitations either in strength or endurance, and so they undertake exploits beyond their capabilities. They draw so liberally upon their balance of vital energy that their account stands in the red. Their extravagance makes them vulnerable to infections and other acute illnesses.

As a teenager you are entitled to ask, How can I tell whether I am as healthy as I should be?

Take a mental inventory of your status. Use the following questions as a guide. If you can answer Yes to all of them, you can be reasonably sure of normal good health. If you have doubts regarding any or must answer No, you should see your doctor and have a checkup.

1. Do you enjoy physical, social and mental activity? It is normal for teenagers to be active. A teenager in good health will be busy from the time he rises in the morning until he goes to sleep at night. If you feel listless or lose interest for prolonged periods in the activities of your schoolmates and friends, then there is reason to make inquiry about your health.

2. Do you recover quickly from fatigue? Every normal teenager gets

## DO YOU

1. enjoy activity, both physical, social, and mental;

2. recover quickly from fatigue;

3. radiate optimism and cheerfulness;

4. make reasonable progress in school;

5. appear healthy with bright eyes, firm skin, and well-developed muscles?

## IF YES, THEN YOU ARE PHYSICALLY FIT.
## IF NO, SEE YOUR DOCTOR.
## IF YES AND NO, CONSULT YOUR DOCTOR.

tired. There is nothing alarming about fatigue which follows activity. A teenager in good health will recover his energy quickly. A brief period of rest or a good night's sleep will suffice when you are in good condition.

3. Are you optimistic and cheerful? If you habitually feel downcast or unusually irritable, you should be concerned.

4. Are you making good progress in school? Of course, some do better than others. Few can expect all A's. What you need to observe is whether you are maintaining your usual position in the class. If your grades have declined recently, or if you seem to have lost interest in school activities, you need help in finding the reason.

5. Is your skin firm, and do you have well-developed muscles? When we speak of a teenager's skin, we recognize that persons of this age often have pimples. Some are particularly troubled with acne. But we are not concerned here with these usual problems. We are interested, rather, in the texture

of the skin. Under favorable conditions, your skin should be firm and ruddy. If your health is impaired, your skin appears sallow, and you tend to scratch and pick at the skin. With respect to muscles, a teenager in good health enjoys activity and develops firm muscles.

### Health Rules for Teens

Suppose you have been able to respond Yes to the five questions. Fine; you are fortunate. But this score does not mean that you should give no further thought to your health. You are in the formative period of life. The patterns you establish now relating to health will persist throughout life. Here are four simple rules that can help you to have continued buoyant health.

*Rule No. 1.* Provide for outdoor physical exercise every day. Most teenage boys need no persuasion on this point. Boys like activity and recognize it as the means of building their muscles. But even though a boy belongs to the ball team at school, it is not probable that the team practices every day. Vigorous exercise once or twice a week does not benefit one as much as exercise taken at least six days of the week.

For the teenage girl, the problem is more difficult. Girls go for feminine skills more than for building their muscles. But they need to reap the advantages of systematic exercise just as much as boys do. A teenage girl will probably become a mother in a few more years. The demands made upon her physical resources by pregnancy, by caring for the young child, and by performing the duties of homemaking will be great. She needs now to build a strong body.

Customarily, modern teenagers follow a way of life that does not require great muscular strength. They ride to and from school. Walking is old-fashioned. They prefer the elevator and the escalator to the stairs. Such customs do not promote physical vigor.

Activities on the playground are

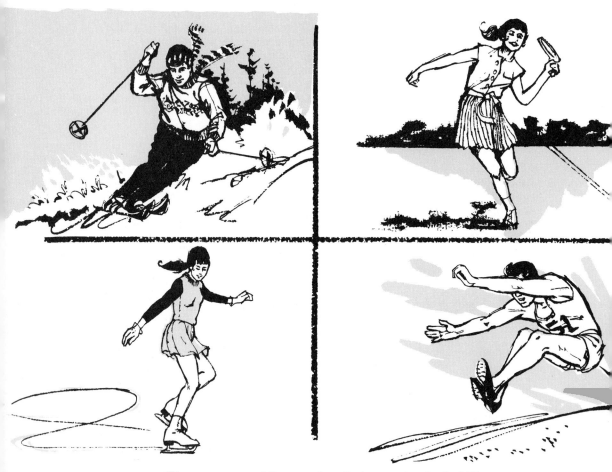

**These are some of the exercises that promote physical fitness.**

good, provided each person gets a sufficient quota of exercise without having to spend too much time idly waiting for teammates to do their parts. It is sustained activity that conditions the heart and lungs and thus increases the individual's vital capacity. Some of the best sustained activities are jogging, hiking, swimming, bicycling, and the use of exercise machines. Weight lifting develops the muscles but does not develop the heart and lungs as effectively as sustained ativities. Of course, productive work requiring the use of muscles rates high as a means of providing wholesome exercise.

*Rule No. 2.* Provide for adequate

sleep. It is during sleep that the body's store of energy is renewed. Restful sleep removes the fatigue that results from the previous day's activities. It restores a person's ability to think clearly. It refurbishes his defenses against disease. A teenager is prone to sleep too little. Bedtime always comes too soon.

A teenager requires more sleep than an adult. Eight hours should be the minimum, and some require as much as nine.

The teenager who stays up late at night to study for tomorrow's examination is only deceiving himself. Having a clear mind while writing the examination the next day will go a great deal farther in guaranteeing a good grade.

See chapter 52, this volume, for additional material on sleep.

*Rule No. 3.* Maintain good habits of eating. Early in the teens, the body grows rapidly—faster than at any other time of life except during the first year. Healthy teenagers are active; and the greater the activity, the more food calories required to provide the necessary energy. In this respect the body is like a machine—it requires fuel to do work; the more work, the more fuel.

A teenager likes food because it tastes good. Also, he likes to spend time in pleasant ways with other teens, both boys and girls. He likes to *do* things, and among his favorite things is eating.

Body weight provides a fairly good index to the adequacy of one's intake. Ideally, girls in their early teens have an average weight of about 110 pounds; in the late teens, about 120 pounds, running a little less for shorter girls and a little more for taller girls.

Boys in their early teens also average about 110 pounds. But boys in their late teens weigh in heavier than girls, at about 140 pounds. Taller boys should weigh more and shorter ones less.

Two prevalent customs prevent teenagers from receiving maximum benefit from their food and so set the stage for poor health: (1) omitting or slighting breakfast and (2) eating snacks throughout the day and evening. The two are related, for when a person does not eat an adequate breakfast he becomes hungry between meals. The ideal plan provides three meals a day, beginning with a good breakfast which includes fruit, an egg or other protein dish, bread, and cereal with milk.

Some teenagers have a weight prob-

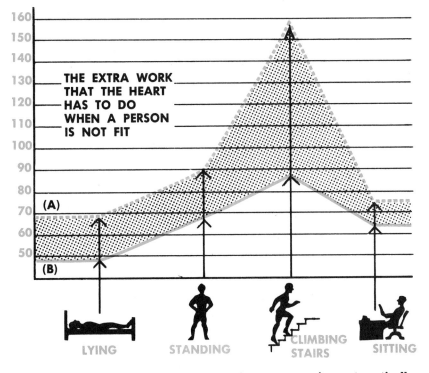

Your heart functions more efficiently when you exercise systematically. The graph indicates the number of times per minute that an average person's heart beats (A) when he has not followed a daily exercise program and (B) when he has exercised vigorously each day.

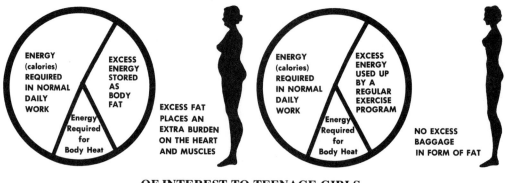

## OF INTEREST TO TEENAGE GIRLS
**It is better to use exercise rather than extreme dieting to keep a trim figure.**

lem. To be really overweight (obese) increases the risks of serious conditions such as diabetes, high blood pressure, and arteriosclerosis, with its accompanying danger of heart attack and stroke. For more on avoiding or correcting overweight see chapter 13, volume 3.

On the other hand, a small group of teenagers actually suffers from undernourishment, even though they live in homes of middle-class status. Strangely, some of these are afraid of becoming overweight, even though their present weight is normal or even less than normal. Teenagers have nutritional needs over and above those of older people, and when they deliberately deny themselves the proper amount of food, they run the risk of reducing the essential constituents of their diet to the danger point.

An illness called anorexia nervosa occurs particularly among adolescent girls in which the individual refuses almost all food. This condition in extreme cases even threatens death by starvation. The girl with this condition seems to be afraid to eat, and so she actually starves herself. She should be cared for by a physician. He will give attention to the amount of food she eats and inquire also into her anxieties and fears to discover why she resists eating. Such a person needs kindly reassurance, plus guidance in following a reasonable program of eating.

Still another group of teenagers attempts to subsist on a diet totally unsuitable. Intake may be sufficient, but much of their food consists of snacks and soft drinks, along with candy and confections. They have just about lost their appetite for good food. The calories they get are "empty calories" because they are short on vitamins, minerals, and other constituents important to well-rounded nutrition.

For further information on the kind of eating habits that promote good health, see chapter 53, this volume.

*Rule No. 4.* Cultivate personal neatness. We do not refer here to a young person's choice of clothes or to how expensive they may be. Neither are we concerned, just now, with color schemes. We are thinking rather of cleanliness and tidiness. We include good grooming because of its influence on self-respect and general health. The well-groomed teenager takes pride in his posture as well as in the way his hair is combed. When he feels well, he walks with chin up and chest out and with a spring in his step.

Personal neatness includes the taking of a shower each day. This habit not only controls body odors but also reacts favorably on the personality to give self-assurance. The daily shower is beneficial to the skin, helping to keep it free from blemishes. When the shower is concluded with cold water, it stimulates the heart and blood vessels, improving circulation.

Personal neatness includes attention to the teeth. Oral hygiene not only improves a person's appearance but goes far in ensuring his future health. The mouth should be rinsed and, preferably, the teeth should be brushed after each meal. We are reminded again of the advantages of a three-meal-a-day program. When a person snacks between meals it becomes almost impossible to keep the teeth and gums free from the fragments of food that make the mouth untidy and that favor disease of the teeth and gums.

### Accidents and Injuries

Accidents top the list of the causes of death among teenagers. Half of these fatal accidents are associated with motor vehicles, the next highest being accidental death from drowning.

Furthermore, accidents leave many survivors permanently handicapped. There are concussions with brain damage; there are bone fractures, many of which heal slowly or leave the victim with a deformity; there are burns (often caused by the explosion of gasoline), which as they heal leave grotesque scars and contractures; and there are cases in which the skin is scuffed away and has to be replaced by skin grafts.

Several reasons account for accident-proneness among teenagers. Teenagers are active and at the same time venturesome. They like to do things exotically different, and often act impulsively.

As a teenager you should recognize your vulnerability in this matter. Keep this risk factor in mind. You need activity; however, take care to choose the kinds of activity entailing the least danger of accident.

You should train well for the kinds of activity you prefer. If you engage in athletics, respect your coach and heed his instructions and the precautions he gives. For other activities, make sure that your developing skill has reached a point of dexterity adequate for dangerous feats. For example, don't swim

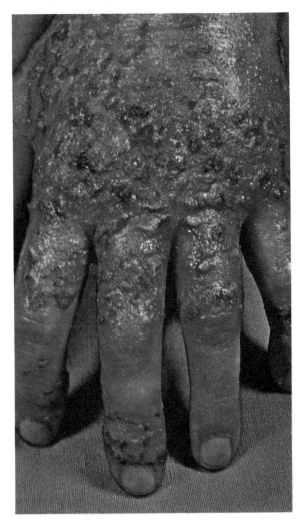

into deep water until you have mastered your strokes in shallow water.

## Skin Disorders of Adolescence

### ATOPIC DERMATITIS (ECZEMA)

The detailed discussion of this skin disease is contained in chapter 17, this volume. There it is mentioned that atopic dermatitis occurs typically in anyone or more of three life periods: infancy, childhood, and young adulthood. We are concerned here with the type that appears during the early teens. It may even last into adult life.

Atopic dermatitis consists of an in-

263

flammatory reaction in the skin characterized by itching, burning, and redness. Its manifestations vary from person to person.

### Care and Treatment

**The teenager with atopic dermatitis will be more comfortable in air-conditioned quarters, for he thus avoids the extremes of temperature which tend to aggravate his skin condition. He will receive some comfort from the use of moist compresses applied to the affected skin areas for one hour, four times a day. The compress consists simply of cotton cloth wrung out of cool tap water.**

**The use of hot water and of soap tends to aggravate the condition. He should avoid these when bathing.**

**Taking a thirty-minute tub bath into which a cup of cornstarch or of powdered oatmeal has been stirred, may help.**

**At times when the skin is not being kept moist by compresses or by tub baths, oil emulsion creams may be used on the affected skin areas. Suitable commercial preparations are Nivea Skin Oil, Lubriderm Lotion, and Keri Lotion.**

**In a more resistant case, the doctor may prescribe a corticosteroid cream to be applied to the involved areas.**

## ACNE (ACNE VULGARIS)

Acne is a common inflammatory disease which affects the skin of the face and, often, that of the neck, shoulders, chest, and upper back. It appears in the early teens and often continues into the twenties. It has been described as the "scourge of adolescence." About 80 percent of teenagers experience some degree of acne, though usually nothing more than troublesome "pimples." Some of these, however—about 20 percent—suffer from the more severe form which leaves scars on the affected skin.

As a child reaches the age of adolescence, the body's glands produce sex hormones which circulate throughout all the body tissues. These hormones

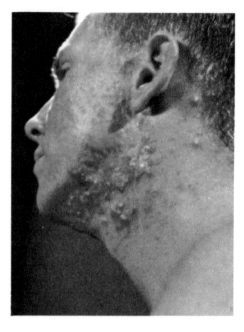

The unsightliness of acne makes it especially detestable to youth.

stimulate the tiny sebaceous glands (oil glands), anatomically a part of the skin's hair follicles. Under this stimulation the cells within a sebaceous gland multiply rapidly—so rapidly that the gland's outlet may become plugged with impacted cells.

The gland continues to be active even though its secretion can no longer reach the surface. As the tiny gland bulges, it stretches the surrounding tissue and produces a small white dot—a "whitehead." Some of the impacted secretion of the gland then undergoes chemical change which causes it to appear black. Thus a typical comedo (blackhead) develops at the site of the hair follicle. As the sebaceous gland and its associated hair follicle are stretched even more, they rupture, producing a local inflammation. In the more severe cases, the breakdown of the delicate tissue permits germs to enter so that an infection develops.

Blemished skin, characteristic of acne, causes the individual to be sensi-

# *Fitness*

A certain natural limit imposes restrictions beyond which the human body does not tolerate carelessness in a person's way of life. It is the purpose of this set of books not only to help you recognize the value of health but to warn you against practices and customs that endanger health and deplete energy, advising you on how to live abundantly, both physically and mentally.

Ask yourself just now, What is it that I want most in life? Contemplate this question for a few moments. Probe into your motives and desires and answer the question honestly.

Perhaps happiness tops your list. Happiness, however, comes as a by-product of good living. Good health and spontaneous vigor enable a person to do the things he enjoys doing. The healthy person is optimistic and cheerful. He can overlook some of the things that would make other people unhappy. If happiness is the first item on your list, you need to cultivate good health.

Or perhaps wealth tops your list. But notice the relationship between good health and wealth. Wealth cannot buy good health, and the person with poor health cannot enjoy wealth. So, if you want to be wealthy, take care of your health, not just to enable you to obtain wealth but to ensure enjoyment of the opportunities that wealth provides.

Or perhaps love tops your list. Love, of course, is a vital influence at all times of life. A child needs the love of his parents. A young adult feels its throb as he searches and finds someone with whom he can share life's choicest blessings. Family members and friends find it to be the mortar which holds together those human relations that enable people throughout life to live abundantly.

But here again notice how important good health is to love. The parent who does not enjoy good health cannot give his child the full measure of love that the child needs. The romance of young adulthood can reach its full measure of satisfaction only as the parties are vigorous and healthy. The personal satisfactions of family life and the delights of friendship are best enjoyed by people with that sparkling vitality that enables them to live unselfishly, employing their energies in the interests of others.

Simple logic, then, makes it clear that maintaining vigor and preserving vitality deserve your sincere and continuous effort. Only as you follow the guidelines of healthful living can you enjoy life to the full—at every stage and in every area of activity and human relationship.

Fitness may be defined as that condition of body and mind which places you at the best advantage as you face the challenges of human experience. Fitness enables you to feel well and to radiate your good feeling. It promotes your resistance to disease so that you will escape many of the illnesses that would otherwise interrupt your chosen activities. It prolongs your life and enriches it with added satisfactions. It enables you to enjoy the rewards of abundant living.

Many factors contribute to fitness. In the present chapter we deal with physical conditioning, (exercise and recreation), the need for adequate restful sleep, the benefits of drinking plenty of pure water, and the importance of mental fitness. The next chapter gives guidelines for selecting a wholesome diet. Then come chapters 54 and 55, which point out the dangers of harmful

**Dwight D. Eisenhower's regular program of moderate exercise markedly prolonged this former President's usefulness to his nation.**

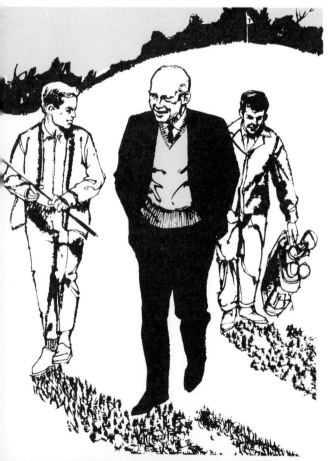

personal indulgences and suggest ways of avoiding popular practices which encourage such indulgences. In chapter 6 advice on maintaining resistance to the infectious diseases by following a plan for immunizations is given. Chapter 13, volume 3, discusses the causes, prevention, dangers, and correction of obesity.

## Physical Conditioning

We sometimes liken the human body to a machine. Both use fuel and produce heat and energy. But obviously many differences exist also, one being the effect of activity.

The potential usefulness of a mechanical device is judged not only by its age but also by how much it has been operated. Use wears it out; and a machine used constantly will wear out sooner than one used only occasionally.

In contrast, the serviceability and life expectancy of the human body is improved by activity. Other factors being equal, the person accustomed to wholesome activity is better off in every way than a person of the same age with sedentary habits.

Anyone physically fit avoids many of the illnesses which handicap others. Body and mind are so interrelated that a physically robust person can use his mind more efficiently. The person is fortunate who from childhood has followed a pattern of systematic physical activity. But even those who have neglected to keep their muscles in tone are not beyond reaping the benefits of physical fitness if only they will now develop a program of conditioning and persist in it.

### Physical Fitness for Youth

We like to think of the period of early adulthood as being the healthiest time of life, and in many ways it is. As yet, the degenerative diseases have not developed. These early years are pace setting for the future.

But it is a sobering fact that many

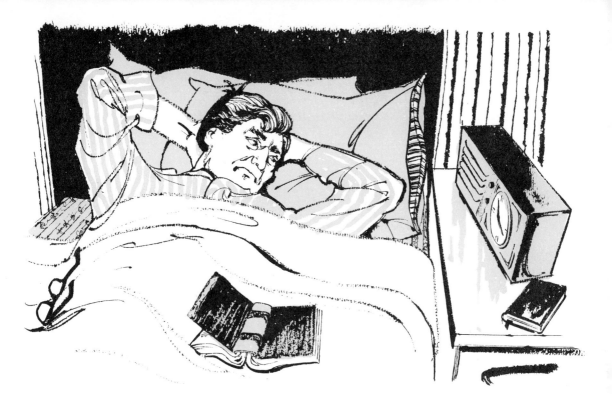

**Distress from not being able to sleep at night may be alleviated by simply putting the mind into neutral and relaxing with the thought that even wakefulness, if quiet and peaceful, can be almost as refreshing as sleep.**

9. Sit or recline quietly for 20 minutes in a bathtub of warm water (not hot) just before going to bed.

10. Arrange your sleeping quarters so as to eliminate distracting noise, bright lights, excessive warmth, or unpleasant odors.

11. Provide a comfortable bed. Once in bed, allow your thoughts to dwell on the comforts of the bed and on your ability to relax. Deliberately allow all your muscles to go slack.

12. If you wake up or lie awake, do not keep track of the time. Persuade yourself that lying quietly relaxed is almost as refreshing as sleeping. Direct your thoughts along peaceful lines.

13. Avoid using sleeping pills or sedative preparations except on a doctor's recommendation. It is better to solve your problems of sleeplessness by removing the cause. The barbiturate

drugs are especially hazardous when used to promote sleep. Their use involves the danger of addiction. Furthermore, no good evidence exists that they improve sleep over the long haul. The same may be said for some of the tranquilizing drugs.

## Abundant Water

We often think of the human body as being a firm, durable structure. This it is, but even so it consists of more than 50 percent water by weight. The body of a person who weighs 154 pounds (70 kg.) contains 40 quarts (40 liters) of water. The fluid portion of the blood consists of water. All of the body's cells contain water. The brain and spinal cord are bathed by a fluid which consists largely of water.

The amount of water which the body

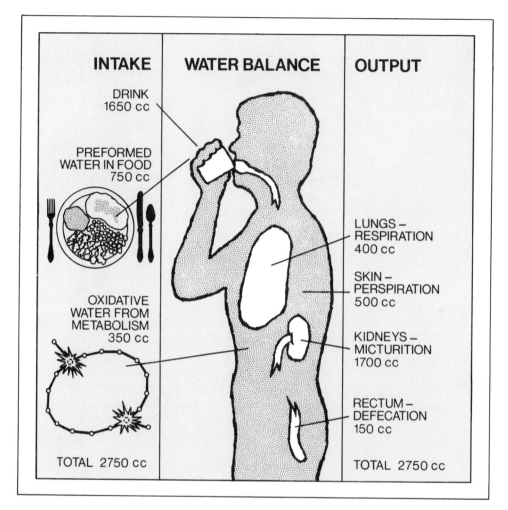

INTAKE | WATER BALANCE | OUTPUT

DRINK
1650 cc

PREFORMED
WATER IN FOOD
750 cc

OXIDATIVE
WATER FROM
METABOLISM
350 cc

TOTAL 2750 cc

LUNGS –
RESPIRATION
400 cc

SKIN –
PERSPIRATION
500 cc

KIDNEYS –
MICTURITION
1700 cc

RECTUM –
DEFECATION
150 cc

TOTAL 2750 cc

**Man maintains the osmotic pressure of his body fluids at optimum level by adjusting his water intake and output. Most of his need of water comes from the liquid itself. Some he draws from the moisture in his food and the remainder he manufactures himself. The importance of this "water of oxidation" varies according to species: the Kangaroo rat, for example, drinks no water at all. His water need, proportionately the same as man's, is met by the moisture in his diet and that which he manufactures himself.**

(Text and adapted drawing © reproduced by permission from *Nutrition Today* magazine, Spring 1970, [P.O. Box 1829, Annapolis, Maryland 21404].)

contains is maintained automatically at a fairly constant level. When an excess is taken into the body, the body retains what it needs and eliminates the rest, mostly through the kidneys in the form of urine. In cases where the body loses more water than it takes in, dehydra- tion develops. Dehydration is a serious condition for adults, but even more serious for an infant.

There are three principal sources of the body's water: (1) the fluid compo- nent of what a person drinks, (2) the moisture contained in the food he eats,

# Choice of Food

The question, What to eat? implies an almost unlimited variety of foods from which to choose. But abundance is one thing; adequacy of diet, another. People usually decide the matter in one of two ways: (1) They eat what they please, or (2) they eat what is best for them. Judging by appearances, most people eat what they please.

Those who eat what they please become slaves to their appetites. If they like a food, they eat it; if they don't, they avoid it. They argue that appetite is a safe guide, and for proof sometimes cite the way animals choose their food.

But examine this contention for a moment. In the first place, animals are not endowed with the degree of intelligence possessed by mankind. A great deal of an animal's behavior is automatic, dependent on built-in instincts. Secondly, specialists in animal husbandry actually do not allow their animals to eat what they please. Instead they determine scientifically what food is best and provide that.

Another observation indicating that appetite is not a safe guide in the choice of food is that it changes with a person's whims. It is easy for anyone to develop an appetite for one food and a dislike for some other. Appetite, being changeable and easily conditioned, is a fickle guardian of health.

Turning our attention now to the second group of people—those who choose their food in the light of what is best and thus make their appetites the servant of their intellect—we must admit that even they may make unwise choices. Before a person can choose wisely, he must know what foods provide the nutritional elements his body needs.

And this observation brings us to the theme of the present chapter—the body's nutritional needs and how best to meet them. Fortunately good food, delightful to eat, may generally be had, plus a constantly growing fund of information on nutrition.

Learning how to eat wisely consists of more than merely memorizing two lists—one of undesirable foods and the other of healthful foods. Eating wisely depends on avoiding extremes in diet, on partaking of a variety of foods rather than on following dietary fads, and on knowing what to include in each day's fare so that the body's needs will be met.

## Characteristics of a Well-nourished Person

Before we get into the details of food selection, we should consider the question, What do we expect of a good diet? A well-nourished individual, provided he exercises regularly and follows a consistent program of healthful living,

tion you face. Merely putting your troubles into words helps you to see new relationships and gives your subconscious mind an opportunity to devise solutions to your problems.

5. *Work off your hatreds.* It is an inborn tendency that makes you want to fight when you become angry. Simply to stifle this tendency does not remove your anger but allows it to smolder in your thoughts. In this frame of mind danger lurks that you will blame innocent persons and that you will pity yourself unnecessarily.

The constructive way to handle anger and hatred is to work it off by physical activity. Chopping wood and beating rugs were the old classic methods. Modern adaptations include playing a set of tennis, spading a plot in the garden, or taking a brisk hike. Just be careful that you don't try to work off your hatred by driving your car pell-mell through traffic!

6. *Learn to be reconciled.* In your effort to succeed, you may have adopted the attitude that things must go your way or else. But the realistic attitude toward life's circumstances requires that you face the fact that you cannot always have your way and that you cannot change some circumstances. When you run into a stone wall, don't keep beating your head against it; find some other more acceptable way of accomplishing what you had set out to do.

7. *Focus on helping others.* A great many harmful tensions stem from selfish attitudes—a desire to have your own way and an effort to keep the other person from putting something over on you.

There is nothing more effective in relieving such tensions than to engage wholeheartedly in some enterprise designed to benefit another person, one for which you will receive no tangible reward. Being neighborly to someone presently in hard circumstances is a move in this direction. Participating in church-sponsored activities will help you to reconcile your personal stresses before they become harmful tensions. Doing a good deed just because it is good for your soul will have the effect of removing pent-up antagonisms.

8. *Trust in God.* If you are a Christian, you have access to the greatest of all aids toward developing a tolerance for life's stresses. The Christian allows the Lord to carry the burden of his trials and perplexities. He trusts God even though it is hard for him to understand the reason why he may be placed in a perplexing situation. He realizes that some good must come from problems not of his own choosing. The Scriptures say, " 'The Lord disciplines those whom he loves; he lays the rod on every son whom he acknowledges.' You must endure it as discipline: God is treating you as sons. Can anyone be a son, who is not disciplined by his father?'' Hebrews 12:6, 7, NEB.

*a.* Milk group:

This group includes milk and milk products, such as cheese, yogurt, and ice cream (used sparingly).

*b.* Protein group:

The group includes nuts, beans, peas, lentils, eggs (not more than 2 to 4 per week), fish, fowl, meat, and meat alternates (analogs).

*c.* Vegetable-fruit group:

A dark-green or deep-yellow vegetable should be eaten at least every other day to ensure adequate vitamin A.

A citrus fruit or other fruit or vegetable should be eaten daily (the reliable source of vitamin C).

Other fruits and vegetables, including potatoes, as desired.

*d.* Bread-cereal group:

This consists of bread and cereals from whole grain, enriched or restored.

3. *Following Planned Menus.* This third method of making sure that the diet provides a nutritionally balanced fare is perhaps of more interest to the homemaker than to other members of the family, for it deals with the planning of meals.

The important point in planning menus is to include during the meals of the day one or more representative items from each of the above mentioned groups. There should not be overconcern in emphasizing any single food or any certain group. A small variety of food each meal, a larger variety per day, and a seasonal variety will provide an acceptable diet.

The accompanying menus provide a pattern of three meals per day: breakfast, dinner, and supper. If your family serves dinner in the evening, use the "supper" menu for the noon lunch, with the "dinner," as listed, being served in the evening.

These menus do not call for any meat, fish, or poultry. If you prefer meat of any kind, then replace the vegetable protein food* (see note in next column) with low-fat meat of your choice.

Following the list of menus for seven days, recipes are given for the pecan patties, the lentil loaf, and the Vegeburger patties listed in the menus.

**First Day**

*Breakfast*
Orange slices
Whole-grain cereal
Linketts*
Hot beverage or milk†
Wheat Toast, margarine

*Dinner*
Sliced tomatoes and avocados
Savory garbanzos (chick peas)
Baked potatoes, margarine
Broccoli with lemon wedges
Tomato juice or something similar
Apple crisp

*Supper*
Low-fat cottage cheese
Large dish of fresh fruit
Soy-and-whole-wheat toast
Peanut butter
Fruit juice or milk

*Note: The vegetable protein foods (analogs) listed in the menus are manufactured by such companies as Loma Linda Foods, Riverside, California, and Worthington Foods, Inc., Worthington, Ohio. Check your market for these products.
† Milk, mainly in low or nonfat form for adults. *Fortified* soymilk may also be used.

**Second Day**

*Breakfast*
Grapefruit
Poached or creamed eggs on whole wheat toast
Blended stewed prunes and apricots
Hot milk drink

*Dinner*
Sauteed chicken-like Soyameat*
and mushrooms
Buttered yams
Green peas
Celery and carrot sticks
Homemade whole wheat rolls, margarine
Lightly toasted mixed nuts

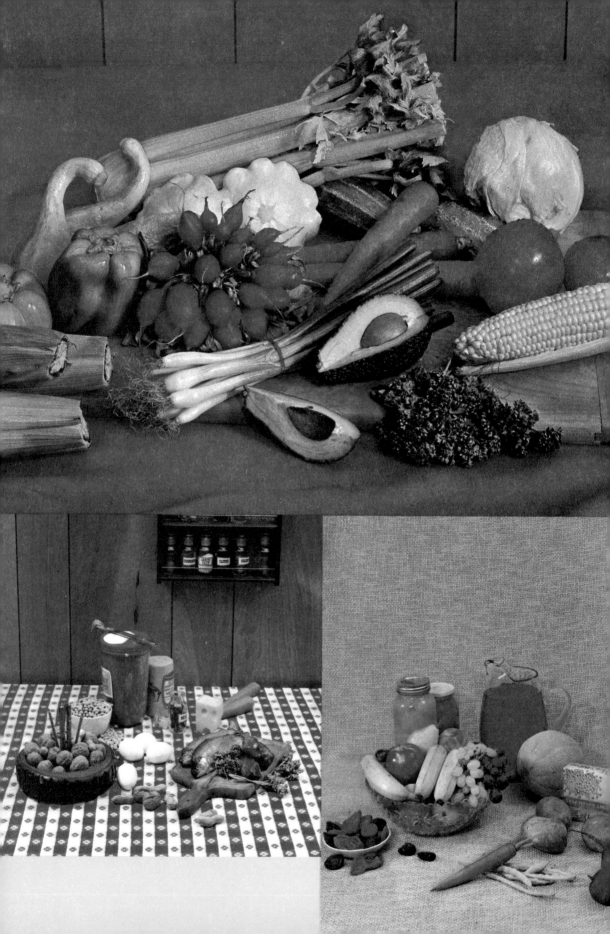

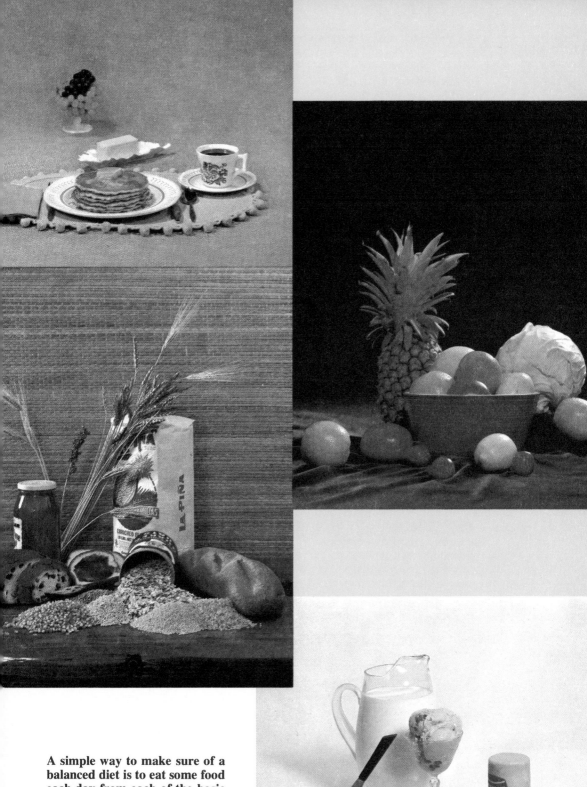

A simple way to make sure of a balanced diet is to eat some food each day from each of the basic food groups. List, page 481.

*Supper*
Cream of tomato soup
Sliced bananas with fresh or
frozen peaches
Corn bread, honey
Buttermilk

### Third Day

*Breakfast*
Orange juice
Soy-and-whole-wheat french toast
with hot berry sauce
Hot malted milk

*Dinner*
Tossed green salad, herb-oil dressing
Pecan patties, brown gravy
Green lima beans
Harvard beets
Sesame-seed rolls with margarine
Date bars
Hot Postum

*Supper*
Toasted Nuteena* sandwiches and
relishes
Mixed fresh fruit bowl
Milk

### Fourth Day

*Breakfast*
Cantaloupe or strawberries
Hashed brown potatoes
Braised meatless breakfast slices*
Breakfast muffins, jam
Hot beverage or milk

*Dinner*
Shredded carrot-and-coconut salad,
pineapple dressing
Navy beans with dumplings
Fresh spinach, lemon wedges
Whole wheat bread, margarine
Oatmeal cookies
Milk

*Supper*
Cottage cheese with peaches
Rye toast, avocado spread
Assorted dried fruits and nuts
Hot Postum with milk

### Fifth Day

*Breakfast*
Grapefruit and orange sections
Hot oatmeal with raisins
Milk
Toasted almonds
Wheat toast, creamed honey

*Dinner*
Baked soybeans in Spanish sauce
Steamed new potatoes
Fresh asparagus spears
Coleslaw with sour-cream dressing
Brown nut bread, apple butter
Milk

*Supper*
Hot Vegeburgers* in whole-wheat
buns
Relishes for buns
Tossed fresh-fruit salad
Hot drink

### Sixth Day

*Breakfast*
Orange slices or cantaloupe
Whole wheat toast with peanut
butter, smothered with hot applesauce
Milk or hot milk drink

*Dinner*
Tomato and avocado wedges with
cottage cheese
Scalloped potatoes
Baked yellow squash
Buttered green beans
Home-made dinner rolls, margarine
Fresh pineapple

*Supper*
Savory split-pea soup
Wheat sticks or crackers
Apricots (canned or fresh)
Milk

### Seventh Day

*Breakfast*
Frozen orange juice
Stewed prunes
Cold whole-grain cereal, milk
Whole wheat toast, nut butter

*Dinner*
Jellied carrot salad
Lentil loaf, brown gravy
Baked potatoes
Fresh peas
Whole wheat rolls, margarine
Lemon pie

*Supper*
Egg sandwiches or meatless cold cuts
Fresh fruit
Hot or cold milk drink

## Recipes

### Pecan Patties

1 1/2 cups uncooked oats
1   teaspoon salt
1   teaspoon sage (scant)
3   eggs
1   cup onions, ground (or 1/2 cup onions and 1/2 cup celery, ground)
1   cup pecans, finely ground

Mix oats, salt, and sage. Add well-beaten eggs, onions, and pecans. Let stand at least an hour; longer if you wish. Form into patties, Brown lightly in a little oil. Cover with thin brown gravy and bake in slow oven about an hour. Makes 6 servings.

### Lentil Loaf

2   cups cooked lentils
1   cup dry bread crumbs
1/2 cup chopped walnut meats
1/2 teaspoon sage
1   teaspoon salt
1   large can evaporated milk
1/4 cup oil
1   egg
1   small onion

Slightly mash lentils. Add dry ingredients. Beat egg, add oil and milk. Add to the lentil mixture. Bake in flat pan in moderate oven for 45 minutes. Cut in squares, arrange on platter. Cover with sauce and serve. Makes 8 to 10 servings.

### Vegeburger* Patties

2   cups Vegeburger*
1/4 cup dry bread or cracker crumbs
2 to 3 eggs, unbeaten
3   tablespoons minced onion

2   tablespoons soy sauce
    Seasonings to taste

Mix and drop by spoonfuls onto hot oiled griddle or skillet. Cook until moisture is almost gone before turning. Makes 8 bun-sized patties.
*See footnote under menu for first day.

### Special Dietary Needs

There are certain times and conditions of life when the average dietary program needs to be modified. The modifications do not involve new patterns of nutrition but only appropriate changes in the basic pattern already described. Seven special situations will be mentioned.

1. *Childhood.* It is during childhood that the eating habits are established. Parents bear the responsibility, therefore, to maintain a home dietary program as nearly ideal as possible. The child thus becomes accustomed to proper nutrition. Eating patterns learned early will guide him all through life in choosing right foods.

A small child does not eat as much, of course, as does a larger child or an adolescent. The proportions of the ideal diet are scaled down to meet a child's needs. He is in a period of growth, however, and must receive an adequate amount of the food elements essential to growth. First among these is milk, vital to the development of bones. In itself milk provides a fairly well-rounded diet, being deficient only in iron and vitamin C. These two deficiencies can be made up by green leafy vegetables for the iron and citrus juice or tomato juice for the vitamin C. A young child should have a cup of milk at each meal, and an older child should consume about a quart a day. More than this is undesirable because it lessens the child's appetite for other foods.

In childhood nutrition it is important to prevent the child from obtaining a large part of his calories from candy and confections. A child soon forms the habit of liking sweet things, and if permitted to draw a large portion of his

485

# *Personal Indulgences*

The body has continuous need for food, air, and fluid. In fulfilling these needs a person supplies his body with the substances essential for life and health. In taking food he provides the materials for energy, growth, and repair of body tissues. In breathing air he brings oxygen to the lungs, from whence it is distributed to all cells of the body. In drinking liquids he provides water, the body's universal solvent and the medium of transportation for life-sustaining elements within the body.

When any of these three substances essential for life are in short supply, internal compulsions develop in the form of hunger, thirst, and a sense of suffocation. These built-in compulsions are safety devices which keep a person from neglecting his body's basic needs.

But in satisfying hunger and thirst, many people have gone beyond the body's fundamental requirements. Influenced by popular customs, they have developed habits to comply with these customs, and have allowed the habits to become cravings. In some cases these additional cravings are for things harmful to the body.

Much of the discomfort and the illness that people experience is caused by careless patterns of living. We therefore highlight the need for preventive medicine—for treating disease be-

fore it occurs by removing or avoiding the conditions that allow disease to develop.

In the present chapter we deal with four indulgences popular in the world today and now condemned by medical scientists for increasing illness and shortening life. We refer to caffeinated drinks, cigarettes, liquor, and marijuana.

## Caffeinated Drinks

### Coffee

Coffee is the favorite hot drink in the United States, as is tea in Great Britain. Almost three million tons of coffee beans are imported, ground into coffee, and consumed in this country each year, an amount equal to about 70 percent of the world's supply. Those who drink coffee dote on its aroma and flavor. Many have preferences for some particular brand. More than half of American adults drink coffee every day.

The taste and aroma alone do not account for the popularity of coffee. Coffee gives a lift which so habituates its users that they feel they cannot perform their usual activities without it. Coffee becomes a crutch on which they depend for a starter in the morning, for a pick-me-up at the coffee break, for

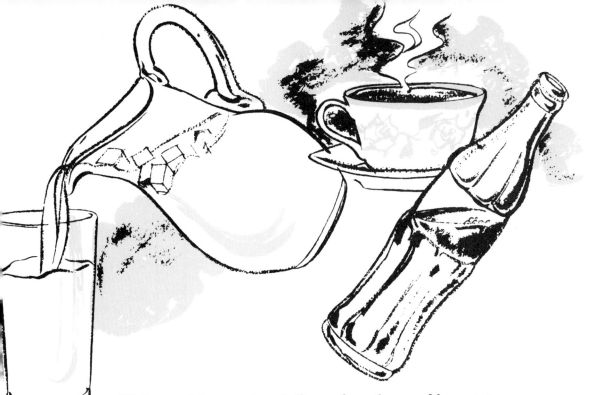

**Wholesome living requires abstinence from the use of beverages detrimental to the body's functions.**

cedure depends upon the body's normal response to exercise and temperature contrast. There is no unfavorable letdown as there is with stimulation by coffee. It is true that in the early afternoon following the exercise and shower of the morning, a person may feel so relaxed that he desires a brief nap. But he does not feel depressed as does the person who craves another cup of coffee.''

Medical literature contains case reports of persons who have suffered from caffeinism, a nervous condition characterized by mild, irregular fever, sleeplessness, loss of appetite, and irritability. It is easily confused with what psychiatrists call anxiety neurosis. It occurs in persons who have been intemperate in their drinking of coffee. In one such reported case, the patient admitted drinking from fifteen to eighteen cups of brewed coffee per day.

Significantly, the symptoms of caffeinism clear up within two to three days after the patient discontinues the drinking of coffee. In one such case the physician persuaded the patient to re-

sume his former indulgence in coffee and, sure enough, the symptoms returned, only to disappear again when coffee drinking ceased.

Scientific studies indicate that coffee drinking is a hazard to the unborn child. Caffeine circulates in the blood of the coffee-drinking expectant mother. It passes through the placenta and enters the blood of the unborn child, where the concentration of caffeine becomes essentially equal to that in the mother's blood. In a series of cases the incidence of spontaneous abortion, of stillbirths, and of premature births was significantly higher in those expectant mothers who drank as much as four to six cups of coffee per day.

In early 1981 a Harvard research team stumbled onto still another indictment against coffee. As reported in the *New England Journal of Medicine,* they found a statistical link between coffee drinking and cancer of the pancreas. Their study found the incidence of the disease, fifth largest cause of

# THE WAYS SMOKING KILLS

An analysis of the deaths occurring among regular cigarette smokers (including those who smoke pipes and/or cigars in addition to cigarettes). Adapted, Hammond and Horn.

| CAUSE OF DEATH | Number of Deaths During the Study | Expected Number of Deaths (had all subjects been nonsmokers) | "Excess Deaths" (above the number expected for nonsmokers) | Percentage of the Total Number of "Excess Deaths" Caused by Individual Diseases |
|---|---|---|---|---|
| Coronary Artery Disease | 3,361 | 1,973 | 1,388 | 52.1 |
| Lung Cancer | 397 | 37 | 360 | 13.5 |
| Cancers Other Than Those Listed | 902 | 651 | 251 | 9.4 |
| Pulmonary Disease (Except Cancer) | 231 | 81 | 150 | 5.6 |
| Cerebral Vascular Lesions | 556 | 428 | 128 | 4.8 |
| Heart Diseases Other Than Those Listed | 503 | 425 | 78 | 2.9 |
| Gastric and Duodenal Ulcer | 100 | 25 | 75 | 2.8 |
| Cancer of Mouth, Larynx, or Esophagus | 91 | 18 | 73 | 2.7 |
| Aneurism and Buerger's Disease | 86 | 29 | 57 | 2.1 |
| Cirrhosis of the Liver | 83 | 43 | 40 | 1.5 |
| Cancer of the Bladder | 70 | 35 | 35 | 1.3 |
| All Diseases Other Than Those Listed | 486 | 453 | 33 | 1.2 |
| Circulatory Diseases Other Than Listed | 87 | 68 | 19 | 0.7 |
| Accident, Violence, Suicide | 363 | 385 | -22 | -0.8 |
| Totals (All Causes) | 7,316 | 4,651 | 2,665 | 100.0 |

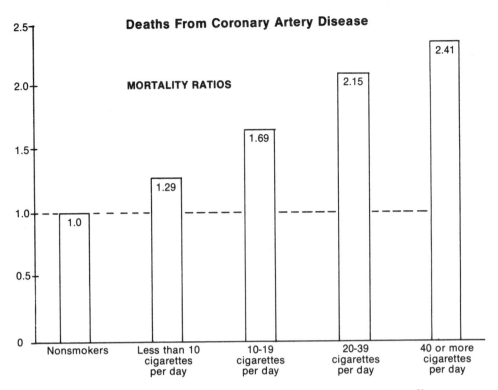

**Deaths From Coronary Artery Disease**

**MORTALITY RATIOS**

Nonsmokers: 1.0
Less than 10 cigarettes per day: 1.29
10-19 cigarettes per day: 1.69
20-39 cigarettes per day: 2.15
40 or more cigarettes per day: 2.41

**Smoking increases the incidence of death from coronary artery disease, with the highest incidence occurring among those who smoke the most. The experience of nonsmokers is used as the standard of 1. (Hammond and Horn study, "JAMA," March 15, 1958.)**

his close friends, this pressure makes it easy for him to succumb.

Third, the impulse to conform. Not only does a teenager want to be accepted by his peers, but he wants to do whatever appears popular throughout the nation as a whole. The tobacco industry capitalizes on this motivation by an extravagant program of advertising, picturing smoking as the "in thing" to do.

A subtle thought sometimes tips the balance in a teenager's thinking, overcoming any reluctance he might have against smoking. He says to himself, "I will try it, and if I don't like it I will quit."

But once a person has a few smokes, he develops a tolerance for the nicotine which cigarette smoke contains. This tolerance is a prelude to addiction.

Ninety percent of established smokers are addicted to nicotine to the extent that they suffer uncomfortable symptoms when the nicotine in their bodies falls below a certain level. So, in order to relieve these symptoms they take another smoke. Starting to smoke, then, is like stepping onto a descending escalator from which it is almost impossible to move upward.

### If You Do Smoke

If you do smoke, consider the health hazards and quit. Quitting is not easy, but it is possible! As previously mentioned, 30,000,000 Americans have quit.

You will not have to wait long before you begin to reap the benefits of quitting. The cough, the excess sputum production, and the shortness of breath

**499**

begin to improve within the first two weeks. Food begins to taste better. Flowers smell sweeter. Just being alive becomes more enjoyable.

What of your susceptibility to the serious illnesses that follow in the wake of smoking? Your body will slowly recover from most of the damage already done. Gradually your prospect of avoiding these serious consequences will also improve, until after a few years your life expectancy will be almost as good as that of nonsmokers.

## Hindrances to Quitting

The smoker who wants to quit does well to recognize in advance the various hindrances he will encounter. Anticipating these, they will not come as a surprise. In the following list of common hindrances, some will apply in one case and some in another:

*Expecting to fail.* Some smokers who try to quit enjoy their smokes so much that they secretly hope they will not be able to quit. They go through the motions of quitting but subconsciously expect to fail in the effort. They almost look forward to saying, "I tried to quit and found it impossible."

*Lack of a plan.* The simple determination to quit is not enough. Smoking has become a part of the smoker's way of life, as firmly integrated into his pattern of living as the style of clothes he wears or the type of recreation he prefers. There must be a studied plan with the details worked out in advance.

*Dependence on nicotine.* It is the nicotine contained in cigarette smoke that produces changes in the way the smoker's organs function. When trying to abstain from smoking, the desire for another smoke becomes almost compelling when the amount of nicotine in a person's body falls to lower levels. Another smoke brings satisfaction because it restores the nicotine level sufficiently to avoid, temporarily, the craving for more. The one-pack-a-day smoker goes through this cycle of crav-

ing and satisfaction twenty times a day—7300 times in a year. No wonder the established habit is hard to break!

*Social pressure.* The smoker tends to be at ease with people who smoke. Once he quits there has to be a reshuffling of his friends. Those who smoke will discourage him in his desire to quit. So there develops an element of loneliness.

*Self-pity.* The smoker has learned to depend on smoking for his personal consolation. It serves him like the infant's pacifier, like the toddler's security blanket. Deprived of smoking, he virtually feels that part of himself is missing. Psychologically, the quitter goes through an experience comparable to grief. It may take weeks to overcome his feeling of bereavement.

*Stressful situations.* When an emergency arises, the first thing the habitual smoker does is to reach for a cigarette. So, in making plans to quit, make sure to select a time that will be as free from stress as possible. Stress automatically triggers the habit patterns that have operated so long for placing a lighted cigarette between the lips.

*Fear of gaining weight.* The recent ex-smoker usually does gain a few pounds. Food tastes better as soon as the taste buds recover from the benumbing influence of cigarette smoke. But gaining a few pounds in the process of quitting is not serious. One challenge to a person's willpower and self-control is enough at one time. Winning the victory over smoking will enhance one's willpower so much that the later problem of controlling weight will not seem so great. It can be taken care of successfully once the major problem of quitting has been surmounted.

*The use of alcohol.* A person who has experienced the effects of liquor and of smoking knows that either one increases the desire for the other. One of the first effects of a drink of alcohol

Our hopes, our destiny, the future of society and of nations, the "Life Stuff by which the human race is perpetuated," as Bernard Shaw once said it, lie folded in the potential growth of children. Boundless capacity for wonderment and guileless response to affection, plus a healthy mixture of mischief, make their own appeal on behalf of a little boy or girl entrusted to the care of parent, teacher, or health guardian.

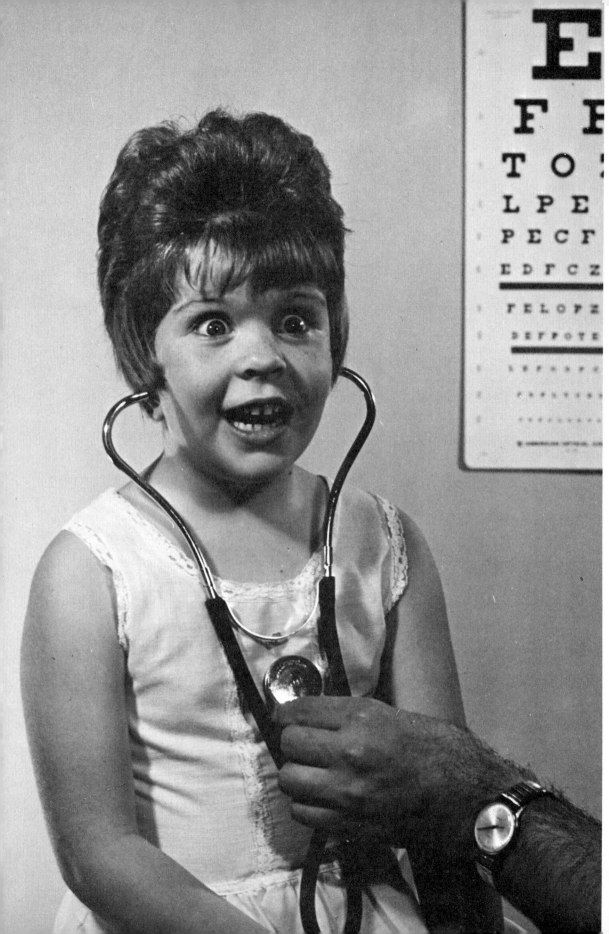

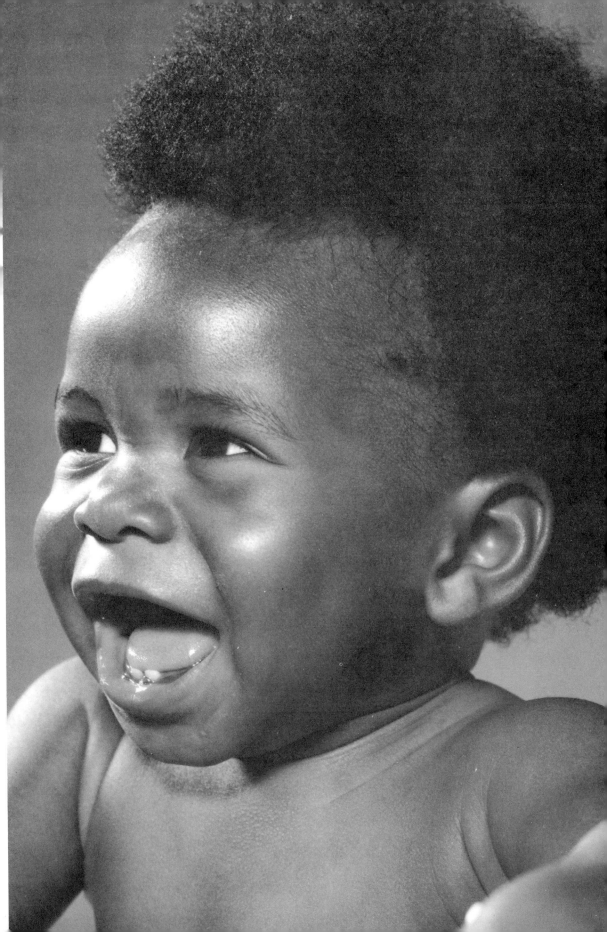

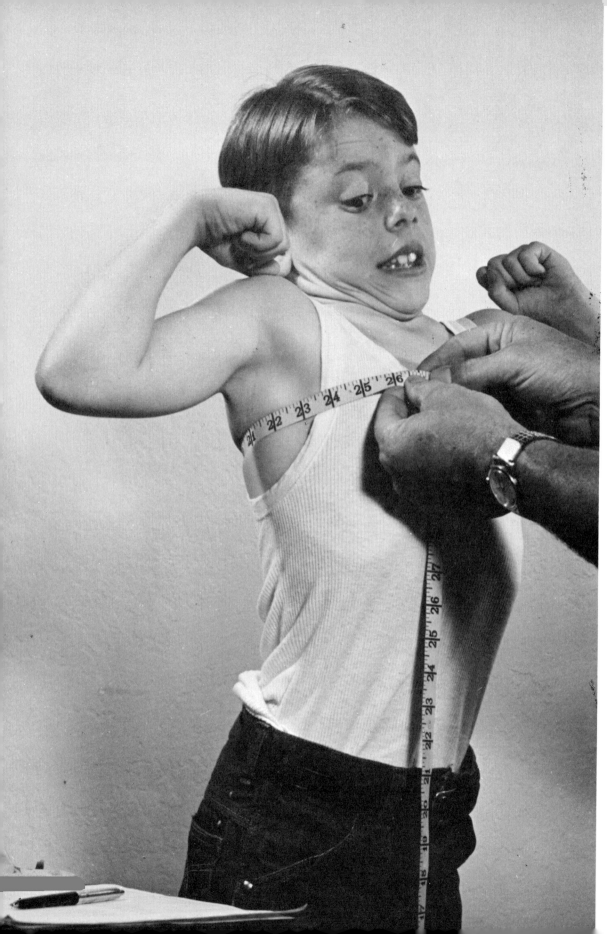

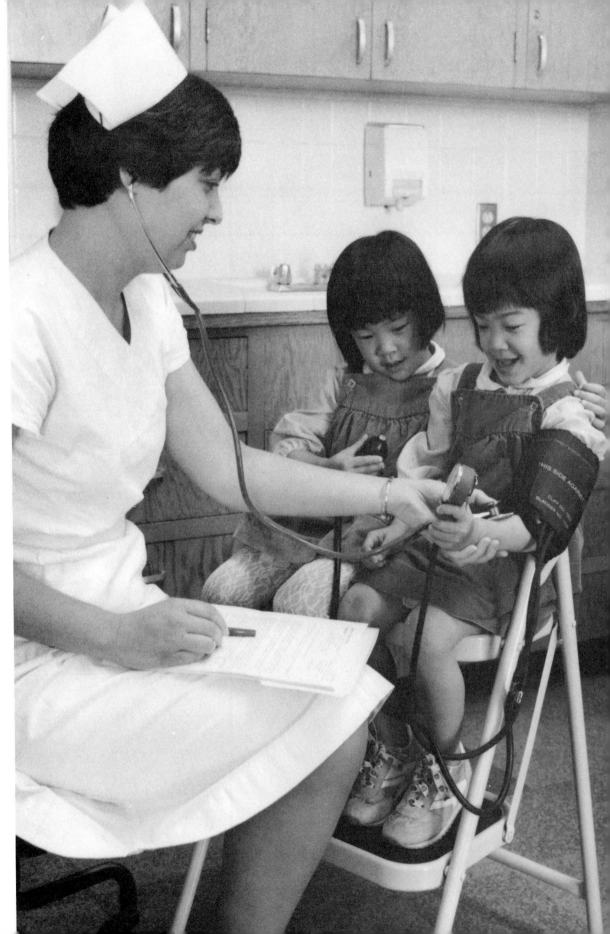

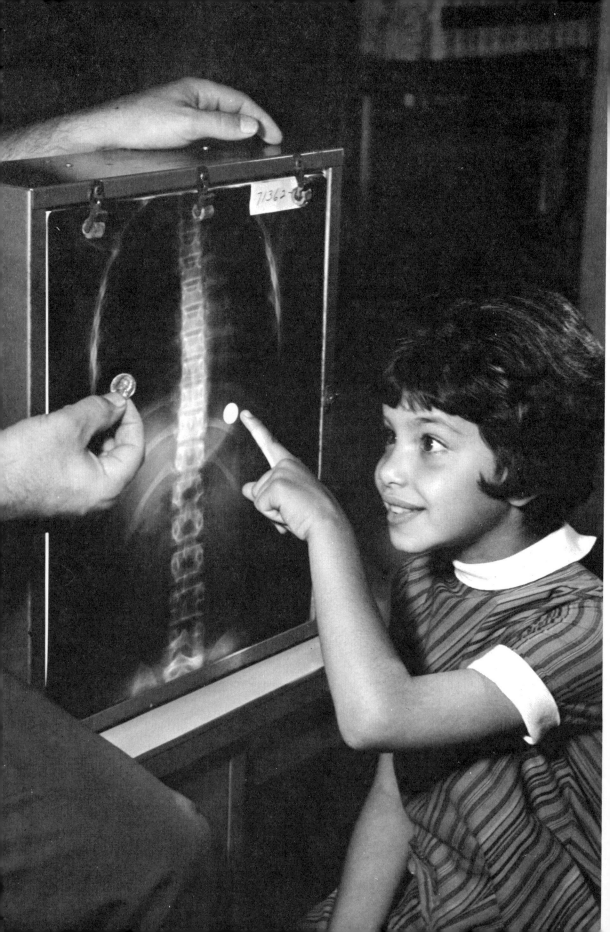

... and help the people to get well too."

# FAMILY MEDICAL RECORDS

Biographical information useful to a physician and others in dealing with a family member's illness and in outlining an individual health-protection program.

## HUSBAND

NAME _____ Date of Birth _____

### CHILDHOOD DISEASES RECORD

| Disease | Approximate age at time of illness | Aftereffects | Doctor |
|---|---|---|---|
| Whooping cough | | | |
| Chicken pox | | | |
| Measles (rubeola) | | | |
| German measles | | | |
| Mumps | | | |
| | | | |
| | | | |

### IMMUNIZATION RECORD

| Disease | Date of immunization | Repeat date | Repeat date | Repeat date | Doctor |
|---|---|---|---|---|---|
| Smallpox | | | | | |
| Diphtheria | | | | | |
| Tetanus | | | | | |
| Polio | | | | | |
| | | | | | |
| | | | | | |

# Drugs: Good and Bad

Drugs are chemicals. Each one is composed of certain kinds of molecules. For the most part, the molecules composing drugs are not the kinds that occur naturally in the body. They intrude into the body's community of molecules and have a chemical influence on the way bodily activities take place.

Many drugs influence the brain. They alter the thoughts, the sensations, the feelings, and the behavior. And this observation brings us to a serious consideration. Inasmuch as some drugs can influence the user's mental activities, a person becomes the victim of the drugs he takes. He trusts part of his very personality to a drug.

Of course if a doctor orders the drug, he takes the responsibility for its effects. But many drugs are sold without a prescription and are more powerful than we realize. The person who chooses on his own to take a drug, takes the responsibility for what happens.

The body has marvelous ways of regulating its own activities. It can adjust to new circumstances. It can respond to stress and to emergencies. It has built-in safeguards. Even pain, as unpleasant as it is, is a danger signal the body uses to call attention to something wrong. Fatigue is the body's way of saying that it needs rest.

Often the real reason for resorting to drugs is impatience with the body's system of safeguards and warning signals. People want to do what they want to do even though it taxes them beyond their body's ability to perform. So they tamper with the body's system of controls and balances by taking a drug to force the issue.

Many available drugs will accomplish the purpose desired. A sleeping pill will put you to sleep. A pain pill will stifle a pain. A tranquilizer will produce a "so what" attitude. And a pep pill or a drink of coffee will seem to release additional energy to keep you going. But you pay a price for these results— too high a price!

A certain drug alters the function of the body in several ways. One way may seem desirable, but other ways may be unfavorable and even damaging. It is because of these harmful side effects that great caution should be used in taking drugs, lest they impair tissues and thus set the stage for poor health and a shorter life.

### Over-the-counter Drugs

Drugstores handle two classes of medicinal preparations: so-called "over-the-counter drugs" and prescription drugs. The former are supposedly harmless preparations available to anyone. The latter, more profound in their

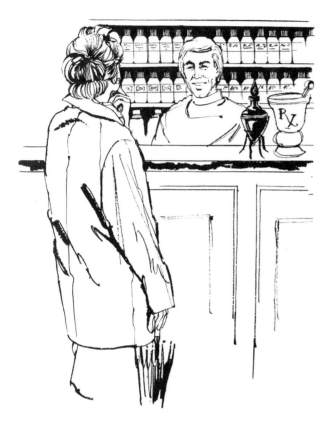

**"Sorry, madam! That preparation can be sold only on prescription from your doctor."**

effects on the human body, are dispensed only on a doctor's prescription.

Aspirin and related compounds account for about one fourth of the drugs sold without prescription. The next largest group consists of remedies for the common cold (including cough drops, syrups, and nose drops), and antihistamines for temporary relief of hay fever.

Vitamins and tonics are also popular at the drug counter. So are laxatives, antacids, and other preparations intended to aid digestion. First-aid preparations and skin remedies make up another substantial segment.

## The Problem of Wakefulness

When nature is unhampered, a person falls asleep at about the same time each night and wakes up about the same time each morning. But certain conditions and events may disturb that pattern. Unhappy with the disturbance, particularly when it keeps him awake, the person may turn to drugs to reshape the pattern more to his liking.

Everyone taking sleeping pills risks three hazards:

*First,* the probability exists of becoming dependent on certain kinds of sleeping pills, the reason being that these kinds contain a barbiturate in one form or another. The person who becomes accustomed to taking a barbiturate finds it increasingly difficult to get along without it. It influences his feelings and reactions. Without it he finds it difficult to relax. He depends on it for sleep. He even feels that he needs it to elevate his mood from mild depression to cheerfulness. And so he takes increasing doses of whatever form of barbiturate he uses. Scientists say that the person thus habituated develops a "tolerance." He may take as much as ten times the amount needed to make an unaccustomed person sleep.

The *second* hazard consists of possible harmful effects on the brain and its functions The heavy user of barbiturates may become sluggish and irritable. He often experiences tremor and other forms of incoordination. He may become mentally confused and even deteriorated. Attempts at this stage to discontinue the use of barbiturates cause serious "withdrawal" symptoms, which include restlessness and anxiety in the daytime and sleeplessness at night. Some persons even experience a few epileptic-like seizures during the several weeks of breaking the drug dependence. Some have hallucinations and delirium.

The *third* hazard is the danger of overdosage. Barbiturates have a way of clouding the memory. Under such influence the person forgets that he has already taken a full dose of the medi-

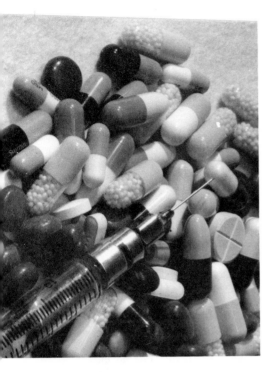

## The Control of Inflammation

Inflammation may be defined as the reaction of living tissues to an injury. It can result from various conditions and circumstances as they affect the body's tissues. It is characterized by swelling, redness due to an increased amount of blood in the injured tissues, increased temperature of the involved tissues, and pain in the area. As a classic example of inflammation, we may cite the condition of rheumatoid arthritis, in which the tissues of the affected joints become inflamed. See the discussion of rheumatoid arthritis in chapter 21, volume 2.

Several drugs tend to reduce inflammation. The salicylates, of which aspirin is the most common example, are reasonably effective. But the salicylate drugs sometimes have unfavorable side effects and should be used with caution. Other drugs more powerful in their effects of relieving inflammation are, at the same time, more hazardous to use because of the more serious side effects they may cause.

Some of the most potent drugs used for combating inflammation are the corticosteroids, first used for such a purpose as early as 1948. Before resorting to these, the physician must weigh the advantage of their use against the prospect of side effects, some of which can be severe and long-lasting.

Certain simple physical agents may also be used in combating inflammation, perhaps the most important being the application of heat to the affected part. This treatment causes an increase in the flow of blood through the inflamed area, helping thus to reduce the inflammation. Resting the affected part of the body is also helpful.

## The Control of Infections

Late in the nineteenth century it was discovered that many infectious diseases are caused by specific germs. People then reasoned correctly that by keeping germs from entering the body they could prevent the diseases pro-

feine contained in coffee and cola drinks. But pep pills are more devastating to the personality. They may produce hallucinations, delusions, mental confusion, and unnatural behavior. These drugs are popularly abused by teenagers.

Cocaine has become quite common among illicit drug users because of the "high" it produces when taken internally. Its proper medicinal use is for producing anesthesia of surface tissues and membranes.

A person pays a high price for the supposed advantage of stimulating his brain to greater activity. It is much better to allow the body's built-in systems of balance and control to regulate one's activities in harmony with personal capacities.

If you crave greater personal efficiency, if you desire to live more abundantly, if you want to be healthy and live longer, don't tamper with pep pills. Build up your physical and mental fitness by living sanely and avoiding excesses.

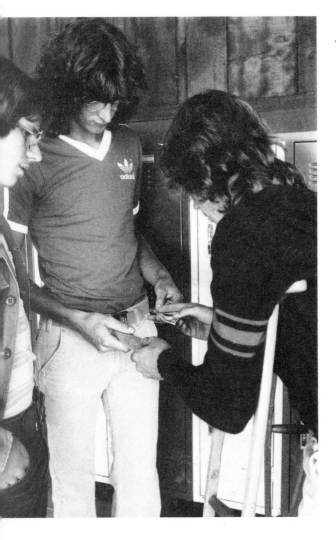

1. *Fear of ridicule by drug-using friends*. The young person who uses drugs usually becomes a member of a group of users. The other members have failed to change their pattern of conduct and they don't want any newcomer to succeed either. They may even be fearful that he would become an informer and make it difficult for the others. Of course, the drug pusher from whom they obtain their drugs will find ways of making it difficult for any of his customers to discontinue.

A teenager needs friends. But it is not easy for the would-be quitter to develop social contacts with those who do not use drugs. So the drug user who desires to reform faces grave problems of social adjustment.

2. *Persisting, unsolved personal problems*. The very problems that prompted the teenager to continue his use of drugs, once he had experimented with them, become more difficult to solve after prolonged indulgence. His use of drugs has weakened his stamina, robbed him of courage, and caused him to lose time in personal development that would have helped him to make advancement.

3. *Fear of failure in life's enterprises*. The chronic drug user is handicapped in obtaining the kind of job he would like to have or in continuing the educational program of his choice. He no longer leads in the competition for good jobs or for scholarships that would enable him to continue school. He feels sensitive about the evidence of his personal failure and so gives in easily to pressures to continue with drugs.

To be successful in helping their teenage child to discontinue his use of drugs, parents must be willing to sacrifice many things. It may be advisable for them to move to another community so that the child will form other friends. The parents should be willing to spend additional time in pleasant companionship with the child. Even if cooperative, the child will still need

the longer he continues his use of them. Somewhere along the line every user becomes aware of the harm drugs are doing him. When not under their influence, he regrets that he started using them and wishes that he might leave them alone.

Some teenagers come to this realization after their first few trials. For them it may be relatively easy to quit. But the longer the individual continues his use of drugs and the greater the difficulty he encounters in solving his personal problems otherwise, the harder it becomes. The real hindrances to recovery may be listed as follows:

# You and Your Health
# Volume 2
# The Human Body
# Diseases
# Symptoms

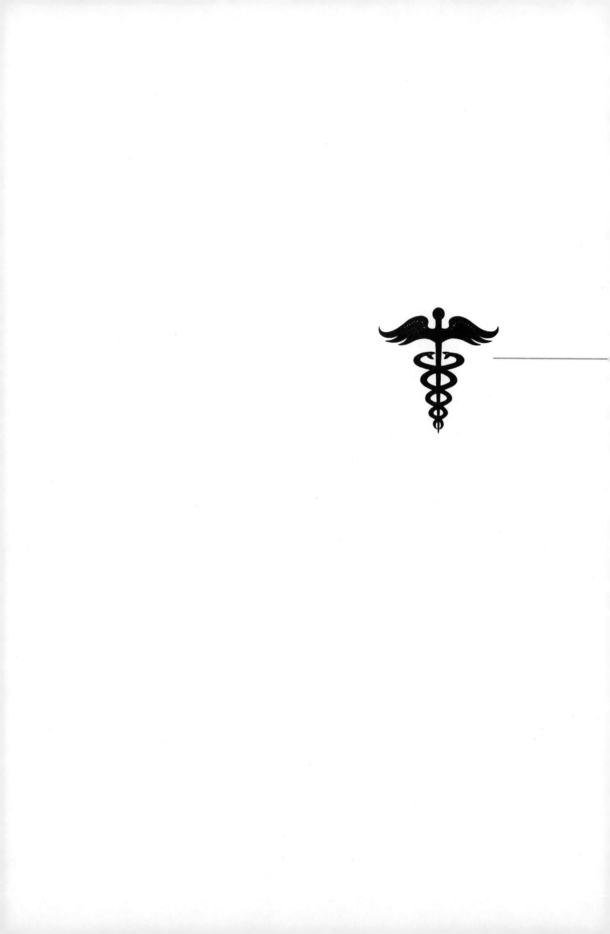

# VOLUME 2
New Edition

You and Your Health

## The Human Body
## Diseases
## Symptoms

## In three volumes, illustrated

Harold Shryock, M.A., M.D., and
Mervyn G. Hardinge, M.D.,
Dr.P.H., Ph.D.
In Collaboration With 28 Leading Medical Specialists

Published jointly by

**PACIFIC PRESS PUBLISHING ASSOCIATION**
Boise, ID 83707
Oshawa, Ontario, Canada

**REVIEW AND HERALD PUBLISHING ASSOCIATION**
Washington, DC 20039-0555
Hagerstown, MD 21740

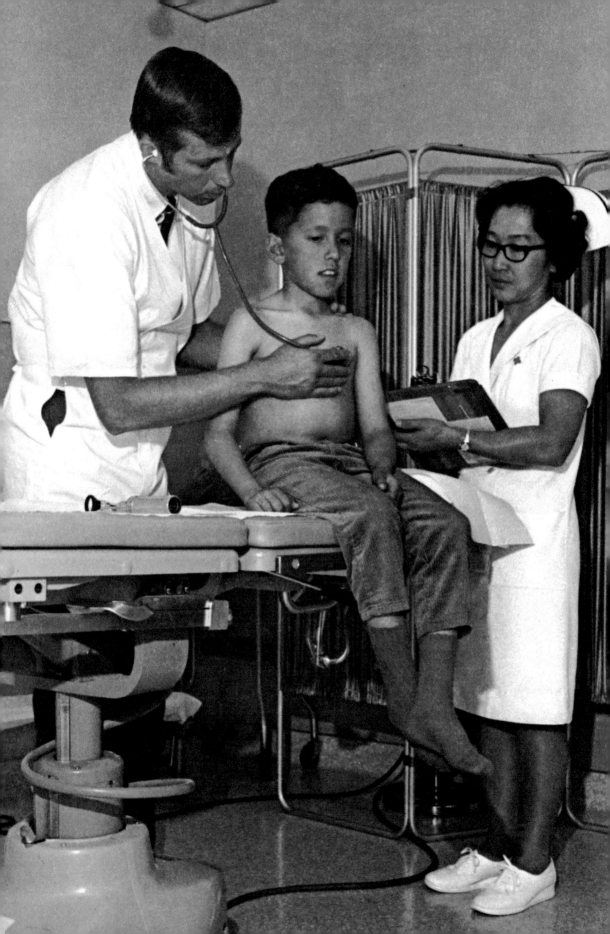

# CONTENTS

# Volume 1—More Abundant Living

SECTION I—Dimensions of Life

Life Has Length, Breadth, and Depth

SECTION II—The Perpetuation of Life

Both Parents Contribute — Motherhood in Prospect — The Child's Development Before Birth — Childbirth — Care of the Infant: in Health, in Illness — Patterns of Growth and Development

SECTION III—On Being Good Parents

The Philosophy of Parenthood — The Father's Part — The Child's Need for Love — Play Activities — Discussing Intimate Matters — Preparing the Child for Life — Hazards of Homelife — The Home's Regulations — Educational and Vocational Guidance — A Child's Problems and Illnesses

SECTION IV—On the Threshold of Adulthood

A New Individuality — Entering Adulthood — Facing Life's Challenges — Relationships With Parents Must Change — Learning to Be Friendly

SECTION V—The Teenager

The Urge to Experiment — How Soon to Love? — Petting, Pregnancy Too Soon, Homosexuality — Teens' Health, Health Problems, and Hazards — Teenage Financing

SECTION VI—Courtship and Marriage

Problems of Courtship — On Getting Married

SECTION VII—Husband and Wife

Respecting Each Other — Differences in Belief — Handling the Money — Dealing With the Children — The Intimate Side of Marriage — Reasons for Tensions — Finding the Trouble — Rising Above Mistakes — Avoiding Divorce

SECTION VIII—Middle and Later Life

Adjusting to Retirement — Illness During Later Life — When Vigor Declines

SECTION IX—Keynotes for Abundant Living

The Tone of Success — The Foundations of Happiness — Personal Maturity — The Knack of Getting Along With People — Rising Above Moodiness — The Control of Temper — Imagination as an Ally — Facing Reality — Mentality: Your Great Asset

SECTION X—Safeguards to Health

Protecting Community Health — Fitness — Choice of Food — Personal Indulgences — Drugs: Good and Bad

FAMILY MEDICAL RECORDS

GENERAL INDEX

# Volume 2—The Human Body; Diseases; Symptoms

SECTION I—Combating Disease

| | | |
|---|---|---|
| 1. Progress in Medicine | | 13 |
| 2. What Your Doctor Can Do for You | | 25 |
| 3. Helps for Diagnosis | | 39 |
| 4. Why Disease? | | 57 |

SECTION II—The Body's Defenses; Symptoms

| | | |
|---|---|---|
| 5. The Marvelous Body and Its Defenses | | 67 |
| 6. Common Problems and Symptoms | | 81 |

SECTION III—The Heart; Circulatory Systems

| | | |
|---|---|---|
| 7. The Heart, Blood Vessels, and Blood | | 111 |
| 8. Diseases of the Heart | | 126 |
| 9. Cardiovascular Disorders; Blood Vessel Diseases | | 141 |
| 10. Blood Diseases | | 158 |
| 11. The Lymphoid System and Related Diseases | | 177 |

SECTION IV—The Respiratory System

| | | |
|---|---|---|
| 12. The Larynx, Air Passages, and Lungs | | 191 |
| 13. Diseases of the Respiratory Organs | | 198 |

SECTION V—The Digestive System

| | | |
|---|---|---|
| 14. The Mouth and Teeth | | 223 |
| 15. Problems of the Mouth and Teeth | | 237 |
| 16. The Stomach and Intestines | | 246 |
| 17. Diseases of the Digestive Organs | | 254 |
| 18. The Liver, Gallbladder, and Pancreas | | 275 |
| 19. Diseases of the Liver, Gallbladder, and Pancreas | | 280 |

SECTION VI—The Skeletal System

   20. The Body's Framework   291
   21. Disorders of the Skeletal Structures   301
   22. Muscles: Their Structure, Function, and Diseases   323
   23. How the Body Derives Its Energy   339

SECTION VII—The Skin and Its Diseases

   24. The Body's Covering   351
   25. Skin Diseases   360

SECTION VIII—Urinary and Sex Organs

   26. The Urinary Organs   405
   27. Diseases of the Urinary Organs   410
   28. The Sex Organs, Male and Female   424
   29. Diseases of the Male Sex Organs   435
   30. Diseases of the Female Sex Organs   444
   31. Sexually Transmitted Diseases   468

PROMINENT ACHIEVEMENTS IN MEDICINE   477
(A Pictorial Supplement)

SELECTIVE ATLAS OF NORMAL ANATOMY   494

GENERAL INDEX   511

# Volume 3—More Diseases; First Aid; Emergencies

SECTION I—The Glands and the Nervous System

The Glands — Endocrine Gland Disorders — The Nervous System — Diseases of the Nervous System — Mental Illness: Neuroses and Psychoses

SECTION II—The Sensory System

The Organs of Sensation — Pain — Diseases of the Eye — Diseases of the Ear, Nose, and Throat

SECTION III—Cancer

Characteristics of Cancer — Manifestations of Cancer

SECTION IV—Dietary Problems

Deficiency Diseases — Disorders of Regulation

SECTION V—Allergies and Infections

Allergic Manifestations — Infections — Viral Diseases —

Rickettsial and Chlamydial Diseases — Bacterial Diseases
— Systemic Fungal Diseases — Parasitic Infections

SECTION VI—First Aid; Poisoning; Emergencies

First-Aid Kits and Home Medicine Chests — Poisonings —
First Aid for Emergencies

SECTION VII—Home Treatments

When Someone in Your Home Is Ill — Simple Home Treatments

HUMAN ANATOMY—"TRANS-VISION" CHARTS

ILLUSTRATED STUDY OF CELLS

GENERAL INDEX

APPENDIX: MEDICAL INFORMATION UPDATE

# Progress in Medicine

Medical science during the last century has kept abreast of civilization's progress and continues in today's jet age to make spectacular advances. Average life expectancy in the United States has increased from 49 years (in 1900) to more than 70 years. This addition has come about largely because control of epidemics and infections has virtually wiped out onetime major killers and because treatment of disease is now based on a knowledge of fundamental causes.

### A Backward Look

Roll back the calendar to 1875. Imagine yourself living back then. What do you see?

Homes are lighted by candles and kerosene lamps. Streetlights burn gas and have to be lighted each evening by the town's lamplighter. There are no telephones. Telegraph is the accepted way to send urgent messages. Typewriters are not yet in general use.

Tuberculosis was the major killer then, causing approximately one out of every five deaths. It affected people of all ages—babies, teenagers, young adults, and oldsters.

At mention of "tuberculosis," we can almost hear some modern schoolboy ask, "What's that?" But in 1875 the word struck terror to many families. Physicians were baffled, for as yet they did not know the cause of the "white plague."

René Laënnec, the inventor of the stethoscope, the instrument that so greatly aided in the diagnosis of tuberculosis of the lungs, had died of this disease at the age of 45. Physicians were more than ordinarily susceptible, it seemed, probably because of their close contact with patients.

Another major health problem in 1875 was infection. A high percentage of the deaths among soldiers in the then-recent Civil War had resulted from germ-infected wounds.

Germs?—Yes, physicians were beginning to read about the work of Pasteur and Koch. Pasteur was beginning to see germs in the microscope, and Koch was learning to cultivate colonies of them in the laboratory. But as yet scientists did not recognize the various kinds of germs, except the rod-shaped organism that causes anthrax and the organisms involved in fermentation as demonstrated by Pasteur. How germs could invade open wounds and then spread throughout a person's body to threaten his life they did not yet understand. (See pictorial supplement at the back of this volume for painting and write-up of Pasteur and six other persons famous in the early and ongoing development of medical science and practice.)

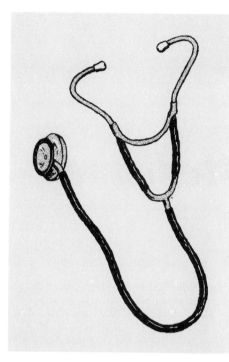

**The stethoscope, invented in the nineteenth century helped immeasurably in the diagnosis of disease.**

In 1875 surgeons wore their street clothes when they performed operations. They carried their instruments in a bag as they went from one patient to the next. The instruments were usually wiped "clean" before being used again, but in doing this, nobody thought of germs.

About 20 percent of the surgical operations performed were amputations, and about half of the patients died of infections that followed. Surgeons shrank from performing operations that required opening of the body cavities. The reason was simple—practically all such cases died of infection even though the surgical procedure may have been done skillfully.

### See What Happened

In 1880, Dr. Edward Trudeau became the promoter in the United States of a revolutionary method of treating tuberculosis. A few years earlier he had cared for a brother who died from tuberculosis. Then Dr. Trudeau developed the disease. The treatment in those days consisted of bleeding, of the application of leeches to draw blood, of blistering of the skin, and of the administration of such drugs as compounds of antimony. Patients were kept in seclusion in dark rooms with no ventilation.

But once Dr. Trudeau became ill he reasoned that if he were going to die, he might as well die happy. Earlier in his life he had spent a few weeks on a hunting trip in the woods of the Adirondacks in upstate New York. Now he determined to return to Paul Smith's hunting camp and enjoy the outdoor life while he lasted. But instead of dying within a few months, Trudeau lived on and even improved. So, as he became able, he resumed his practice of medicine, specializing now in the treatment of tuberculosis by encouraging a way of life which promoted the patient's resistance to the illness.

In 1882 the germ that causes tuberculosis was identified. In 1896 the X ray came into use and since then has been a great help in the diagnosis of tuberculosis and in following either the progress of the disease or the progress of the cure, as the case might be.

By the 1940s and 1950s surgical methods were in use by which one lung, when affected by tuberculosis, could be collapsed so that it could rest while healing took place. But the big breakthrough came with the availability of isoniazid, often used in combination with other drugs. It stifles the growth of the germs that cause tuberculosis.

Notice what has happened. From being a major killer in 1875, by 1900 tuberculosis had dropped into second place as a cause of death in the United States. By 1937 it was in sixth place. By 1950, in seventh place. And now it is not even listed among the major causes of death. But tuberculosis still occurs, with about 30,000 new cases registered each year and about 5000 deaths.

A similar, remarkable improvement

# What Your Doctor Can Do for You

It is natural and customary for every family and sometimes individual persons to have certain selected professional people that they go to for help as needed. A man has "my barber," and a woman has "my hairdresser." A family has "our pastor," and a husband and wife have "our banker." A businessman has "my lawyer." So it is logical that every family have "our doctor," and every single person have "my personal physician."

Now that medical science has developed in so many directions, doctors specialize in the various fields of medicine and surgery. Each specialist is trained and experienced in his own field, such as in the treatment of skin diseases, in problems relating to bones and joints, in the diagnosis and treatment of disorders of the endocrine glands, or in disorders of the nervous system.

But a family does not want a specialist as the family doctor. Rather, they need someone interested in the family's total well-being. It matters not what a person's ailment may be, the family doctor must be one who either treats the specific illness himself or helps to arrange an appointment with a physician who specializes in the treatment of the problem.

Time was when we spoke of personal physicians as "general practitioners of medicine." These were physicians who had completed the regular medical course and had become licensed as physicians, but had not chosen to take additional training in a specialty. People tended to regard these general practitioners as less qualified for diagnosis and treatment than those who had become specialists. But the picture has changed.

Medical educators and people in general have come to realize that the family doctor needs to be as fully qualified in the general field of medical science as does the specialist need to be well informed and experienced in his limited field. And so there has developed the profession of "family practice."

This "specialty" dates back to 1969 when the American Board of Family Practice was officially established. This professional organization supervises and certifies a period of training (usually three years) beyond the regular medical course for those physicians who select family medicine as their professional field of choice. The training of such a physician includes instruction and experience in handling emergencies, guidance in hospital procedures, supervision in common surgi-

# SUGGESTED SCHEDULE FOR PERIODIC CHECKUPS

| Procedure | Value | Frequency |
|---|---|---|
| **A. FOR INFANTS** | | |
| 1. Search for congenital defects and endocrine disorders | To provide for early treatment as indicated | See chapter 6, volume 1 |
| 2. Establish a plan for immunizations | To protect the child against infectious diseases | See page 35 in this chapter |
| **B. FOR CHILDREN** | | |
| 1. Review schedule for immunizations | To maintain protection against infectious diseases | At age 5 and 15 |
| 2. General physical examination | To detect abnormalities or illness | At age 3 and 5 and every 3 years thereafter |
| 3. Blood count and urinalysis | To detect anemia or kidney disease | At age 3 and 5 and every 3 years thereafter |
| 4. Check hearing and vision | To correct and avoid handicap in school | At age 3, 5, and 8 |
| 5. Check teeth | For referral to dentist as needed | At age 3 and 5 and every 3 years thereafter |
| 6. Check blood pressure | To detect beginnings of high blood pressure | At age 5 and 15 |
| **C. FOR ADULTS TO AGE 39** | | |
| 1. General physical examination of heart, lungs, skin surface, and all body openings | To provide clues for beginning illness and to discover need for corrective procedures | Every 2 to 3 years |
| 2. Check blood pressure | To detect beginnings of high blood pressure and to check on the heart's general function | Every 2 to 3 years; oftener if abnormal |
| 3. Pap smear for women | To provide information on the general condition of the uterus, cervix, and vagina, and to signal the possible beginning of cancer | Every year for 2 to 3 years; if favorable, then at 3-year intervals |
| 4. Electrocardiogram (EKG) | To detect changes in heart function and to provide a basis for comparison in later years | At age 35 |
| 5. Skin tests for tuberculosis | When there is a positive test after previous negative tests, further search should be made for the site of a tuberculous infection | Every 5 years |
| 6. Tests for venereal disease | To provide opportunity for treatment even in the absence of symptoms | Every 2 to 3 years for sexually active persons |

| Procedure | Value | Frequency |
|---|---|---|
| **D. AGE 40 AND THERE-AFTER** | | |
| 1. General physical examination of heart, lungs, skin surface, and all body openings | To detect beginning disease and indicate the need for corrections | Every 2 to 3 years |
| 2. Check blood pressure | To detect the beginnings of high blood pressure and to check on the general function of the heart | Every 2 to 3 years; oftener if abnormal |
| 3. Sigmoidoscopy | This examination of the last portion of the large intestine provides a clue to the beginning of cancer in this area | Every 2 to 3 years |
| 4. Blood count and urinalysis | To detect anemia or kidney disease | Every 2 to 3 years |
| 5. Chemical blood tests | A check on the cholesterol level helps in determining the risk of arteriosclerosis; elevated blood sugar may indicate diabetes; level of urea nitrogen indicates kidney function; and level of calcium in the blood is a check on parathyroid function | Every 5 years |
| 6. For women: physical examination of the breasts plus X ray (mammography) if lumps are present | These examinations by a physician supplement the woman's self-examination as a clue to cancer | Every 2 to 3 years; oftener if lumps are noted |
| 7. For women: pap smear examination | To indicate the condition of the uterus, cervix, and vagina, and to signal the beginning of cancer of the cervix | Yearly for 2 years; then every 2 years, but oftener if abnormal |
| 8. For men: prostate examination by palpation | For detection of beginning cancer | Every 2 to 3 years; oftener if abnormal |
| 9. Stool examination for ''hidden blood'' | To check on the possibility of cancer or other bowel problems | Every 2 to 3 years |
| 10. Check on hearing and vision | To indicate the need for referral to specialists in these fields | Every 5 years |
| 11. Tonometry | This simple measurement of pressure within the eye can indicate beginning glaucoma and its threat to vision | Every 2 to 3 years; annually if family history of glaucoma |
| 12. Electrocardiogram (EKG) | To indicate the quality of the heart's function | Every 10 years; oftener if abnormal |
| 13. Immunizations for pneumonia and flu | To protect against illnesses which are serious for older persons | Every year for senior citizens |

YOU AND YOUR HEALTH

### The Physician as a Health Counselor

Many of the diseases which cause suffering and premature death can be avoided if the factors in the environment or in the individual's life-style which cause these diseases are eliminated. And this observation brings us to a recognition of the importance of a physician's influence in helping his patients to avoid the factors that make them susceptible to disease.

Patients should feel free to ask about things that perplex them. Physicians realize, more and more, their responsibility to help their patients understand the principles of healthful living. It is at the occasion of the periodic examination, as described in the previous section, that the patient and his doctor have the best opportunity to consider these matters of healthful living.

Physicians as now trained for family practice have a knowledge of the various risk factors that make persons susceptible to illness. For example, the most frequent cause of death among men in their prime of life is coronary

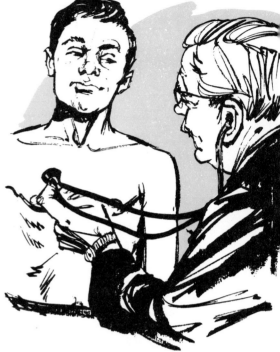

Do youth need periodic checkups? See accompanying schedule.

## CAREFUL EXAMINATION CAN DETECT THESE AND OTHER ——— DISEASES BEFORE THEY PRODUCE SYMPTOMS ———

*Heart disease—various kinds
*High blood pressure and hardening of the arteries
*Cancer:   of the breast
           lung
           stomach
           colon
           rectum
           uterus
           skin
Lesions of the rectum and lower bowel
Anemia
Kidney disease
Diabetes
Tuberculosis
Glaucoma

*The first three on this list are today's "major killers." Valuable time can be gained and lives can be saved by discovering and treating them early.

ease, see chapter 17, volume 3.

4. *Q Fever*. This disease somewhat resembles pneumonia and occurs commonly among persons who have close contact with domestic animals or animal carcasses. It is relatively common in the southwestern part of the United States.

There is a vaccine available to protect against Q fever. However, the vaccine causes local reactions in some of those who receive it. It is therefore recommended that the vaccine be used only for persons at high risk of this disease, such as dairy workers, wool sorters, tanners, and slaughterhouse workers.

For a further discussion of this disease and the accepted treatment, see chapter 17, volume 3.

5. *Pneumococcal Pneumonia*. Various germs and viruses can cause pneumonia, one of the most common being the pneumococcus bacterium, of which there are 14 strains. In 1968, there was released for use a polyvalent vaccine which is effective in protecting against this type of pneumonia. Its use as a preventive measure is recommended for elderly people and those with serious chronic diseases. The protection offered by the use of this vaccine lasts for three to five years.

For a further discussion of the various kinds of pneumonia, see chapter 13, this volume.

### When You Travel

Several serious contagious diseases prevail in certain parts of the world but not in others. These include cholera, epidemic typhus, yellow fever, typhoid fever, and plague. When a person travels to areas where these diseases occur, it is imperative, of course, that he be protected in advance. Travel agents and public-health officials can give advice on the particular immunization procedures to be followed and for what countries.

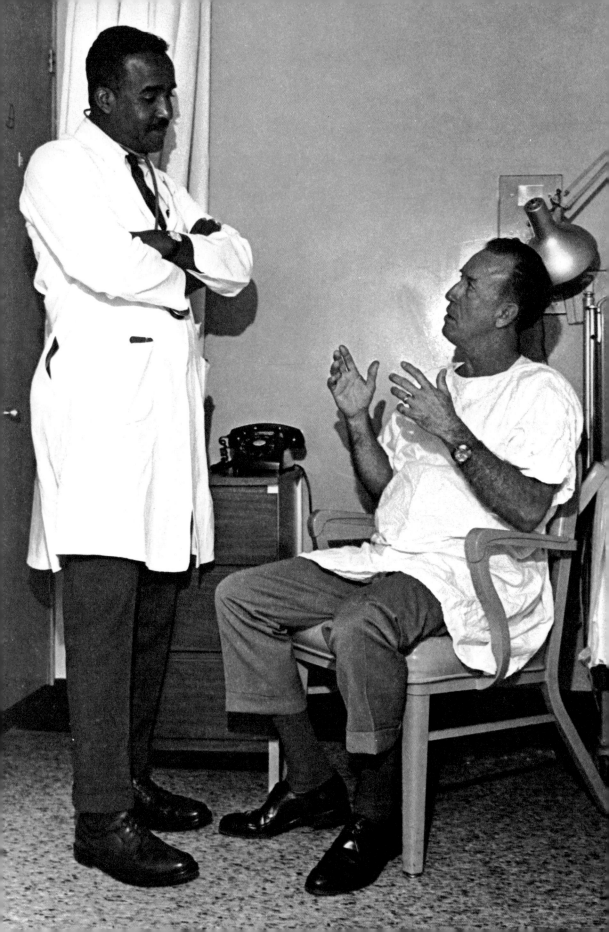

# The Heart; Circulatory Systems

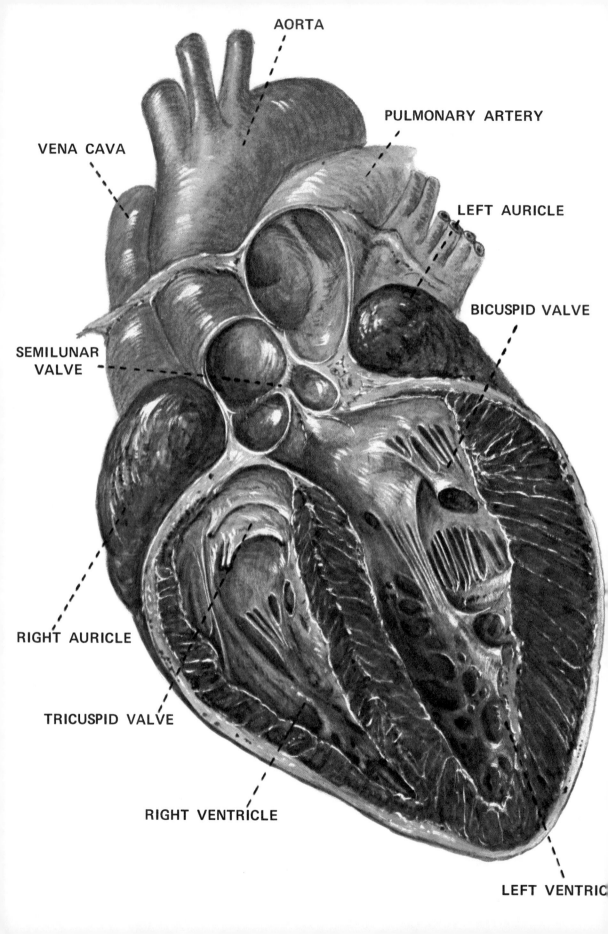

AORTA

PULMONARY ARTERY

VENA CAVA

LEFT AURICLE

BICUSPID VALVE

SEMILUNAR
VALVE

RIGHT AURICLE

TRICUSPID VALVE

RIGHT VENTRICLE

LEFT VENTRIC

# The Heart, Blood Vessels, and Blood

In an earlier chapter the body has been called a living machine. It can be compared to a steam or gasoline engine. It uses fuel and produces heat and power, needing oxygen from the air in order to do so. The chief fuel it uses is blood sugar (glucose), which comes from food. Also, somewhat like an engine, the body sometimes needs repair materials. These also come from food. Waste materials results from the activities of the body, just as smoke and ashes or exhaust gases are produced by an engine.

The classes of food needed by the body, both for fuel and for repairs, and how these are changed by the digestive organs and the liver into forms that can be used by the body tissues will be discussed later. But in this chapter we are concerned with two questions: (1) How are the fuel and repair materials and the oxygen carried to the tissues throughout the body where they are needed? (2) How are the waste materials transported from the tissues where produced to the lungs and kidneys to be discharged from the body? Obviously neither the fuel nor the repair materials are produced *where* needed for use. And just as understandably, the wastes, if they were to remain where produced, would soon clog the body

machine and bring it to a dead stop. So both cases require transportation.

The answer to both questions is the same: The job is done mainly by the blood. The blood, the vessels through which it flows, and the heart which propels the blood through the vessels form the main parts of the body's transportation system.

### The Heart

The heart is about the size of a clenched fist. In the average man it weighs about ten ounces (400 grams), and in the average woman about eight and a half ounces (350 grams). Its walls are thick and composed almost entirely of heart muscle. As this muscle contracts, it squeezes the blood from inside the heart out into the arteries. The arteries then carry the blood away from the heart to all parts of the body.

The body of an adult man of average size contains about six quarts (5.4 liters) of blood. The blood, pumped by the heart, is constantly on the move. Ordinarily a drop of blood can make one complete trip from the heart to some distant part of the body and back again in about one minute. When a person is exercising, his blood can travel even faster. It is remarkable how the heart keeps on year after year perform-

**111**

ing the work necessary to keep the blood circulating without wearing out.

The heart does an enormous amount of work. If you were to lift a ten-pound weight three feet off the floor every thirty seconds (about the same as lifting a four-kg. weight to a height of one meter), you would be doing as much work as your heart regularly does. It would be quite an undertaking to lift this weight this high two times a minute for an eight-hour day, but the heart keeps up its work hour after hour and day after day for an entire lifetime. On the average, the heart of an adult pumps more than 4,000 gallons (14,400 liters) of blood each day.

One reason that the heart is able to carry its heavy workload is that it rests briefly between beats. Studies of electrocardiograms (scientific records of the heart's activities) indicate that the organ's rest periods add up to more time than its working periods. Another reason is that the heart's own tissues

have a very excellent blood supply. Weight for weight, the heart's tissues receive about five times as much blood as the average of other tissues in the body. The heart uses about one tenth of all the oxygen used in the body. Still another reason is that this organ has remarkably great reserve power. For a short time in an emergency, it can do ten times as much work as it has to do while the body is at rest.

The arteries which carry blood into the walls of the heart are called *coronary* arteries. It is important to keep all the arteries in as healthy a condition as possible, but especially these. Doing so is largely a matter of proper diet and proper exercise. Diet is discussed in chapter 53, volume 1. But the chief points to mention here are as follows: (1) the advisability of limiting fats, and (2) the advantage of avoiding obesity by moderation in eating. As to exercise, the ideal is to engage in enough brisk exercise *every day* to stimulate

**The position and relative size of the heart.**

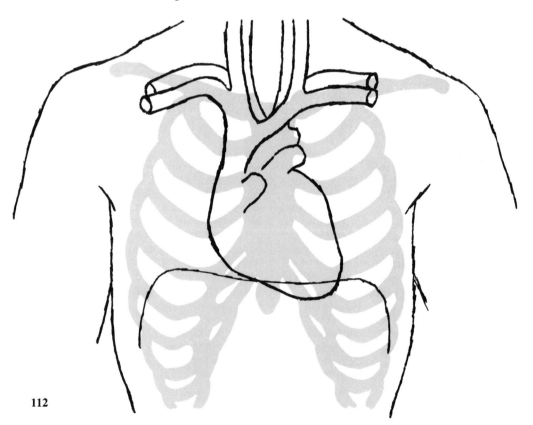

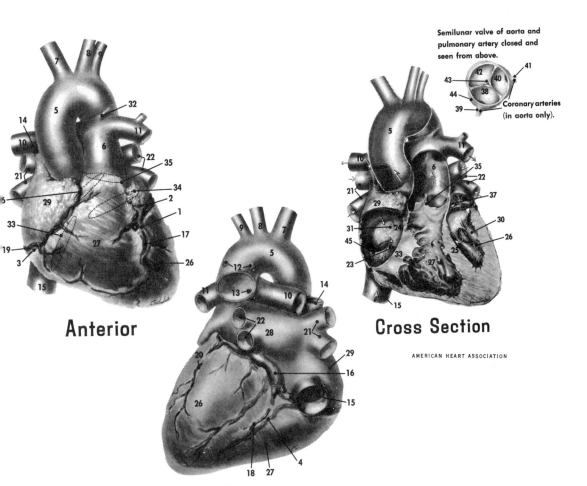

**Anterior**

**Posterior**

**Cross Section**

Semilunar valve of aorta and
pulmonary artery closed and
seen from above.

Coronary arteries
(in aorta only).

AMERICAN HEART ASSOCIATION

## Three views of the heart, showing relative position of its parts.

1. Anterior interventricular branch of left coronary artery
2. Circumflex branch of left coronary artery
3. Right coronary artery
4. Posterior interventricular branch of right coronary artery
5. Arch of aorta
6. Pulmonary trunk
7. Brachiocephalic artery
8. Left common carotid artery
9. Left subclavian artery
10. Right pulmonary artery
11. Left pulmonary artery
12. Posterior intercostal arteries
13. Bronchial artery
14. Superior vena cava
15. Inferior vena cava
16. Coronary sinus
17. Great cardiac vein
18. Middle cardiac vein
19. Lesser cardiac vein
20. Posterior vein of left ventricle
21. Right pulmonary veins
22. Left pulmonary veins
23. Opening of coronary sinus
24. Limbus of fossa ovalis
25. Interventricular septum
26. Left ventricle
27. Right ventricle
28. Left atrium
29. Right atrium (shown opened on cross-section drawing)
30. Posterior papillary muscle
31. Fossa ovalis
32. Ligamentum arteriosum
33. Tricuspid valve (anterior cusp of left valve shown on cross-section drawing)
34. Mitral valve
35. Pulmonic valve
36. Aortic valve
37. Left coronary artery
38. Right valvule of aortic valve
39. Right coronary artery
40. Left valvule of aortic valve
41. Left coronary artery
42. Posterior valvule of aortic valve
43. Nodule
44. Aortic sinus
45. Valve of the inferior vena cava

113

but not to overwork the heart, with due regard to the person's age and previous exercise habits. Exercise is discussed at length in chapter 52, volume 1.

Sometimes in older people the coronary arteries become diseased and unable to carry their usual amount of blood. Such deterioration is serious because it deprives the heart muscle of its quota of blood sugar and oxygen. Sometimes disease of the coronary system causes an artery to become plugged up suddenly. This sudden loss of blood to a part of the heart's wall may cause the heart to lose its efficiency. This is the cause of death in cases of fatal "heart attack."

Each side of the heart contains two chambers. The chambers of the right side receive the blood which comes back from all parts of the body. This blood is brought to the heart by two large veins. One vein, the superior vena cava, brings blood from the head and arms. The other, the inferior vena cava, brings blood from the body and legs. The blood in these veins has already given up most of its supply of oxygen and is loaded with carbon dioxide.

Coming in through the large veins, blood first enters the upper chamber called the right atrium. (See accompanying diagram.) The right atrium sends the blood on into the right ventricle, which has a valve at its inlet and another at its outlet. The inlet valve keeps the blood from flowing backward into the right atrium. The outlet valve keeps the blood from flowing back into the right ventricle after it has been pumped out into the pulmonary artery.

The pulmonary artery and its branches carry the blood from the right side of the heart to both of the lungs. In the lungs, the blood exchanges its load of carbon dioxide for a new supply of oxygen. The blood is then carried by pulmonary veins to the left side of the heart—first to the left atrium, from which it passes to the left ventricle. The left ventricle has more heart muscle in its wall than any of the other chambers of the heart. This is needed

because the left ventricle must pump very forcefully in order to send blood out to all parts of the body. The left ventricle has a valve controlling its inlet and another controlling its outlet, which work much like the corresponding valves of the right ventricle.

### The Heart Sounds

When a doctor listens to your heart through a stethoscope, he hears it beating in rhythmic fashion. The heartbeat gives a double sound which is classically described as lubb-*dup*. After this double sound, there is an interval of quiet and then the lubb-*dup* occurs again: lubb-*dup*—lubb-*dup*—lubb-*dup*. The "lubb" sound is produced by the closing of the valves between the atria and the ventricles. That is, when the

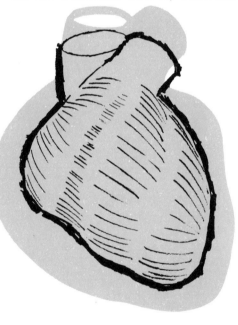

**As muscular wall of heart contracts, the size of the heart changes.**

ventricles begin to contract, the increased pressure causes the blood in them to back up against their inlet valves and close them. As the ventricles continue to contract, they force the blood in them out into large arteries—the pulmonary artery and the

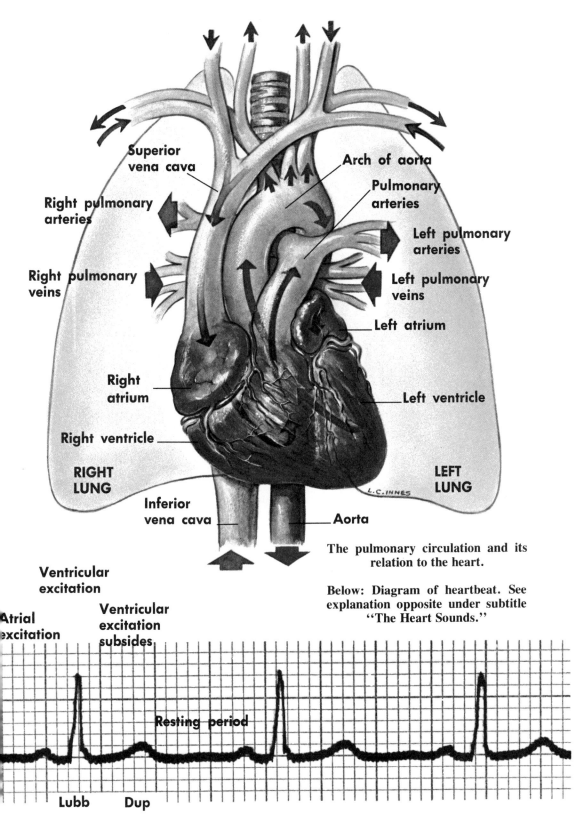

**Superior vena cava**

**Right pulmonary arteries**

**Right pulmonary veins**

**Right atrium**

**Right ventricle**

**RIGHT LUNG**

**Inferior vena cava**

**Arch of aorta**

**Pulmonary arteries**

**Left pulmonary arteries**

**Left pulmonary veins**

**Left atrium**

**Left ventricle**

**LEFT LUNG**

L.C.INNES

**Aorta**

The pulmonary circulation and its relation to the heart.

Below: Diagram of heartbeat. See explanation opposite under subtitle "The Heart Sounds."

**Ventricular excitation**

**Atrial excitation**

**Ventricular excitation subsides**

**Resting period**

**Lubb**    **Dup**

aorta. Then as the ventricles relax in preparation for their next contraction, the blood which has been forced out into the arteries backs up against the outlet valves, closing them. It is the close of the outlet valves that accounts for the *"dup."* It is during the interval between one lubb-*dup* and the next that the heart rests.

### Arteries, Capillaries, and Veins

The left ventricle pumps its blood into the aorta, which is the body's largest artery. The aorta branches so as to carry blood to all parts of the body. The branches of an artery are smaller, of course, than the parent vessel. Finally the branches become so tiny that the blood cells have to pass through them in single file. These very smallest blood vessels are called capillaries. There are many billions of capillaries in one person's body. If they were placed end to end to make a single tube, the capillaries from one adult's body would reach more than twice around the earth.

**Cross section of the artery and the small vein. A. Artery. B. Vein. a. Muscular membrane much thicker in artery than in vein. b. Internal membrane. c. External membrane.**

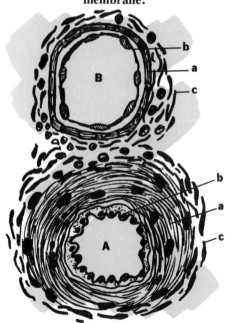

The walls of arteries are composed largely of smooth muscle and elastic connective tissue. This allows for considerable change in the caliber of these blood vessels and, as naturally follows, for considerable change in the amount of blood which can flow through them. The need for such a change will appear more clearly as this discussion continues.

The walls of capillaries are composed mostly of a single layer of endothelial cells. They are so thin that oxygen and food substances pass through easily.

The capillaries do not have either smooth-muscle tissue or elastic fibers in their walls, so they do not change much in caliber. But they can be taken out of, or put back into, service as the needs of the tissue require. The more active the tissue, the greater the number of capillaries in service. When a tissue is relatively inactive, capillaries take turns, in relays, as they care for the tissue's transportation needs. The mechanism of control by which certain capillaries rest while others continue to carry blood is probably by a selective contraction of smooth muscle in the walls of the small arteries at the junction between artery and capillary.

As soon as the blood has passed through the capillaries it starts on its way back to the heart. All vessels that carry blood toward the heart are called veins. The walls of veins are much thinner than the walls of arteries. These walls also have smooth muscle and elastic fibrous tissue in them, but less of it. In a healthy body all the veins are carrying blood all the time, but sometimes they may be almost collapsed and at other times fully distended. Their walls can stretch enough to enable the veins to carry back to the heart all the blood that the arteries and capillaries can bring to them.

Most veins have small valves built into their walls. These valves tend to keep the blood from flowing backward. As you exercise, your muscles squeeze the veins, and the blood inside them is caused to move toward the heart.

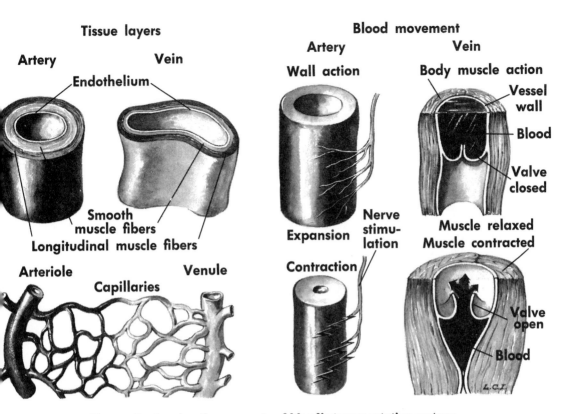

**Composite showing three aspects of blood's transportation system: tissue layers of artery and vein; movement of blood through artery and vein; the capillary system.**

Then, as your muscles relax, new blood flows in to fill the veins again. This is another reason why it is important to keep your muscles in good condition by taking daily exercise. When your muscles act, they help your blood to move faster on its way toward the heart.

As a barber stands quietly by his chair, the blood in the veins of his legs tends to stagnate. Because he is in a standing position, the blood is not easily lifted back up to the level of his heart. The weight of this column of blood gradually stretches the walls of the veins in his legs until the valves cannot close properly. A vein thus stretched and enlarged is called a varicose vein. (See more on this in chapter 9, volume 2.) Not only barbers but other people whose work requires them to stand for long periods in one location, should make it a point to sit down or lie down occasionally, or to walk about a bit when they can during their working hours, as a means of helping to keep their leg veins in good condition.

### Blood Pressure

The arteries of the body have thicker walls than the veins. Larger arteries have thicker walls than small ones. These walls must be thick because the blood as it leaves the heart is under high pressure. The pumping action of the heart is what builds up the pressure of the blood. This pressure is necessary in order to force the blood quickly to all parts of the body. At each beat of the heart, the arteries are stretched a little as they receive a new quantity of blood. You can feel the pulsation caused by each beat of your heart by pressing your finger over the radial artery in your wrist (on the thumb side of the wrist). Counting the pulse at the wrist is the usual means by which a doctor or nurse can tell how fast the

117

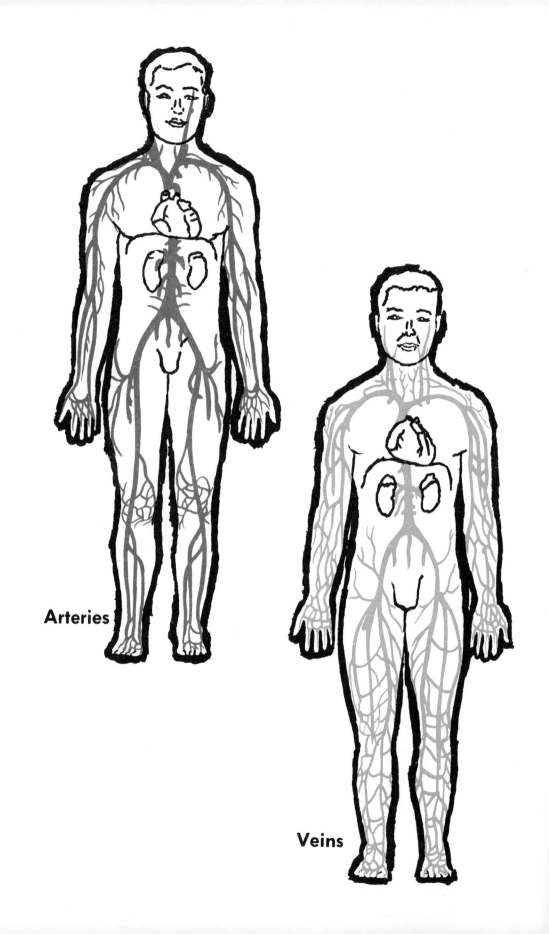

Arteries

Veins

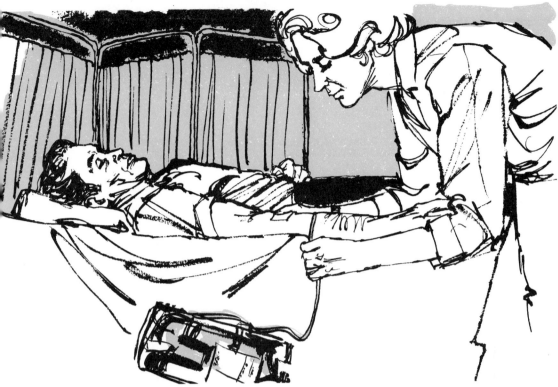

**Human donors are the only source of blood for
patients needing transfusions.**

stored in blood banks for emergencies. The average adult can give about one pint (450 ml.) of blood at a time without endangering his health, provided he does not do so too often.

### Conclusion

Having given so much attention to the fluid part of the body's transportation system, let us briefly reconsider where this fluid goes, what it picks up or unloads at each station, and what happens to the cargo. Parts of this story have already been told in this chapter. That is, blood comes to the right side of the heart through two large veins: one from the upper part of the body and the other from the lower part. Next it goes to the lungs, and then comes back again to the heart, but this time to its left side. Then it goes through the aorta and its branches to all parts of the body,

and back again through the two large veins to the right side of the heart.

When the blood arrives at the right side of the heart, it is carrying carbon dioxide and other wastes which it has picked up in the tissues. When it arrives in the lungs, it unloads its carbon dioxide and picks up oxygen, but keeps its other wastes. When it leaves the left side of the heart and arrives at the tissues, it unloads the oxygen and picks up a new load of carbon dioxide, and also picks up more of the other wastes.

So far as carbon dioxide and oxygen are concerned, this is all of the transportation story. But think a moment. What about other wastes? And what about the food materials that the tissues need? During every circuit, part of the blood goes through the skin and part of it through the kidneys. The skin throws off a small part of the wastes in

# Diseases of the Heart

More people suffer and die from heart disease than from any other ailment. One out of every eight adults in the United States has some form of heart ailment. Some forms of heart disease strike suddenly, causing premature death or invalidism. Others allow their victims to linger for years with reduced vitality.

It is coronary heart disease—the one that causes the typical "heart attack"—that accounts for the greatest number of deaths from heart disease. We will give coronary heart disease its proper emphasis later in the chapter.

## CONGENITAL HEART DISEASE

The heart develops very early in the life history of a human being. At about three weeks after conception, the heart consists of a single tube which pulsates. It is during the next five weeks (weeks 3 to 8 following conception) that the heart becomes a four-chambered organ. The wonder of it is that it is able to continue pumping blood while still undergoing the marvelous transformation from a simple tube to a four-chambered organ.

Considering its complex plan of development, it is not surprising that mishaps occur from time to time which result in malformations of various features of the heart and of the large blood vessels. About nine out of every thousand babies born have some deformity of the heart or the large vessels adjacent to it.

There are many types of congenital heart disease, and the degree of handicap from these varies from person to person. Many cases can be greatly improved and lives extended by modern heart surgery.

For a more complete discussion of congenital heart disease see chapter 17, volume 1.

## RHEUMATIC HEART DISEASE

Rheumatic heart disease is a serious complication of rheumatic fever. As discussed in chapter 17, volume 1, rheumatic fever often follows an attack of streptococcic sore throat or some other form of streptococcal infection. Once a child has had rheumatic fever, the probability exists that he will have other attacks from time to time. Suitable preparations of antibiotics help to prevent these recurring attacks.

During an attack of rheumatic fever there is a strong possibility that the heart will become inflamed. This may take the form of (1) *endocarditis* (inflammation of the lining of the heart or of the valves), (2) *pericarditis* inflammation of the covering of the heart), or (3) *myocarditis* (inflammation of the heart muscle).

A streptococcic infection such as

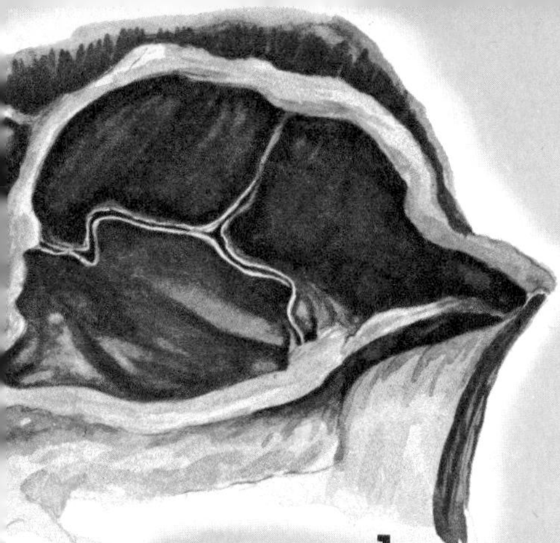

**1**

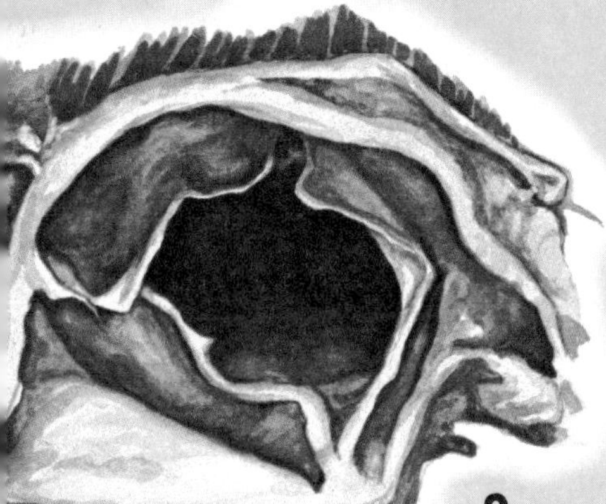

**2**

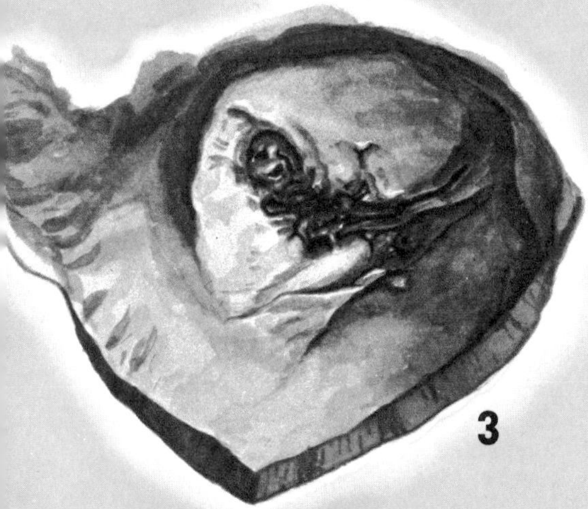

**3**

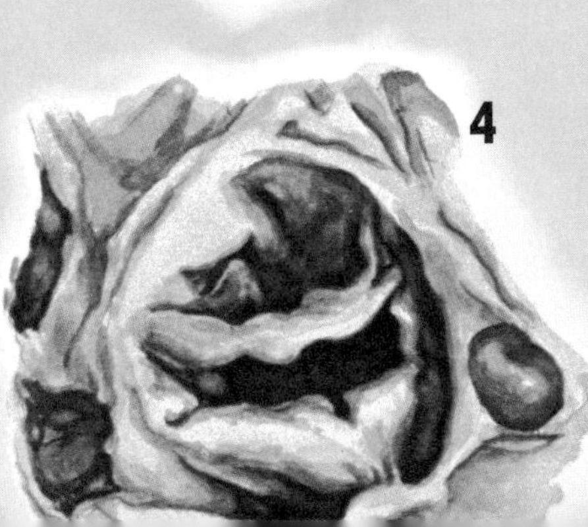

**4**

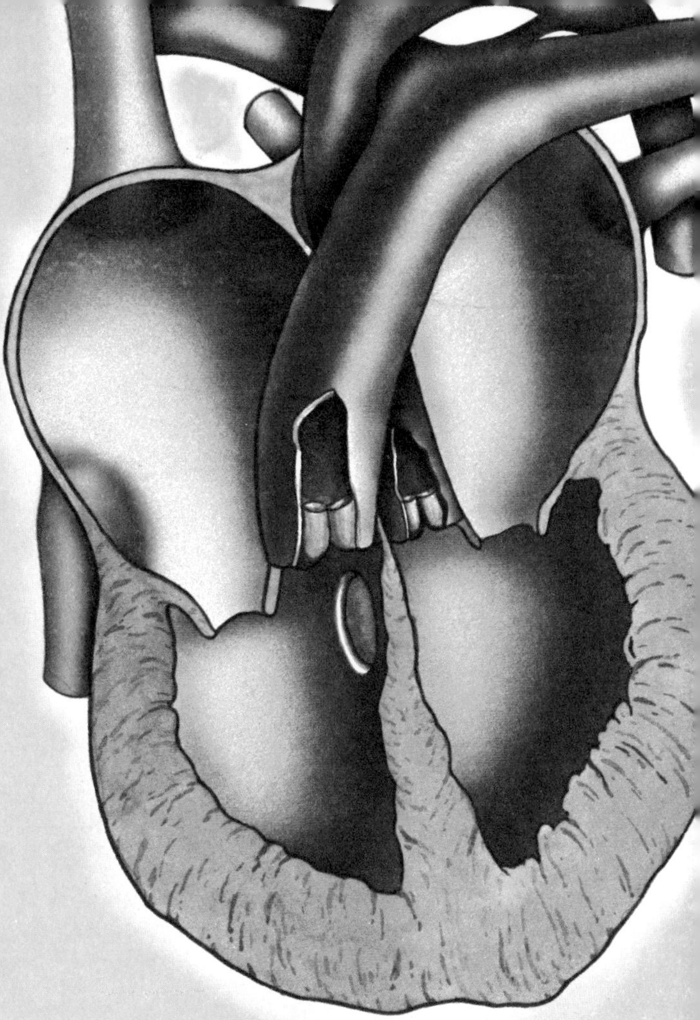

Left: Inflammation in connection
with rheumatic fever may damage
the heart valves. (1) Normal aortic
valve closed. (2) Normal aortic valve
partially open. (3) The mitral valve,
showing narrowing of valve opening
(stenosis) caused by scar formation.
(4) Damaged aortic valve.
Above: Congenital heart defect,
showing abnormal opening in the
wall between the right and left sides
of the heart.

127

streptococcal sore throat does not always produce a typical case of rheumatic fever. Such an infection may cause damage to the heart without passing through the stage of rheumatic fever. Thus, the prevention of rheumatic heart disease requires prompt and adequate treatment of all streptococcal infections when they occur. Once the heart becomes thus involved, there is danger of permanent damage to its tissues.

The valves of the heart are delicate structures covered on each surface with the heart's lining membrane. The inflammation of endocarditis typically causes ulcerations of the valves. As the acute stage gradually passes and the ulcerations heal, two defects may result: (1) a narrowing of the valve opening caused by scar formation and (2) an incompetency of the valve because its leaflets no longer fit perfectly when they contact each other. A narrowing of the valve opening is called stenosis. An incomplete closing of the valve, which permits some of the blood to flow in reverse direction, constitutes insufficiency. The valve more frequently affected by rheumatic heart disease is the inlet valve of the left ventricle (the mitral valve).

### Care and Treatment

Once the valves of the heart have become damaged, the heart's efficiency may be so reduced that it can no longer keep up with the demands upon it. This deficiency may result in disturbed functions of the heart such as atrial fibrillation or in so-called congestive heart failure, both discussed later in this chapter.

Inasmuch as rheumatic heart disease is a complication of rheumatic fever and inasmuch as rheumatic fever is caused by an infection by the streptococcus germ, the treatment consists essentially of combating the streptococcal infection. This requires the aggressive and continuing use of antibiotic medications as prescribed in chapter 17, volume 1.

In the chronic phase of rheumatic heart disease, which may continue into adulthood, it is advisable to consider surgical repair or even the replacement of a damaged heart valve. Physicians specializing in diseases of the heart and in heart surgery should be consulted.

## INFECTIVE ENDOCARDITIS (BACTERIAL ENDOCARDITIS)

Infective endocarditis is a serious disease which, if untreated, is uniformly fatal. The essential feature of the disease is the establishment of a colony of germs in some area of the lining of the heart. The disease was formerly called bacterial endocarditis because the colony of germs that becomes established within the heart was thought to consist always of bacteria. It is now recognized that in occasional cases the infection may be caused by fungi or other disease-producing germs.

There are two types of infective endocarditis, acute and subacute. The acute type is caused by more aggressive, more virulent germs and, if untreated, will run a course of not more than six weeks before causing death. The subacute type is caused by organisms which are more leisurely in producing tissue damage, which cause milder symptoms, but which are just as deadly in the long run as those which cause the acute form of the disease.

*Predisposing Circumstances.* In order for infective endocarditis to develop, there must first be germs in the blood (bacteremia). The germs then lodge in the delicate tissue which lines the heart (the endocardium). If, for any reason, the endocardium is already blemished, the germs establish at the blemished sites. Such blemishes may consist of (1) congenital defects, (2) heart valves that were damaged by some previous illness (as rheumatic fever), or (3) scars from previous heart surgery. But there are cases of infective endocarditis in which the heart's lining was normal and still a colony of germs lodged there. These are cases (as

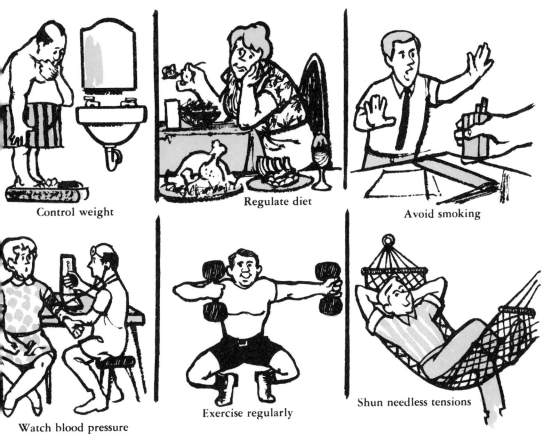

Control weight

Regulate diet

Avoid smoking

Watch blood pressure

Exercise regularly

Shun needless tensions

**Safeguards against heart trouble.**

occurred. Modern methods of examining the coronary arteries have indicated, however, that spasm does actually occur, even to the extent of reducing significantly the amount of blood carried to the heart muscle. There may be several causes for these attacks of spasm of the coronary arteries, among them being the psychological stress of unsolved problems and the use of cigarettes.

We have mentioned that when the heart muscle does not receive its necessary quota of blood, symptoms develop. The symptoms consist of varying degrees of discomfort, sometimes extreme discomfort, in the central chest, in the arm (most often the left arm), and sometimes in other parts of the body. It is this type of discomfort that constitutes angina pectoris. The reader should note that we have not used the word *pain* in describing this symptom of distress. Some patients with this type of discomfort use the word *pain*, but others describe it as a feeling of pressure. At any rate, in a typical case, the discomfort is extreme and causes the patient to discontinue whatever physical activity has caused the heart to be in short supply of blood.

The symptoms of angina pectoris may be brought on by emotional shock or even by a bad dream in which the person's body reacts as to some sudden emergency. It is in such cases that the basic cause of the discomfort is probably a spasm of the coronary arteries rather than a narrowing because of arteriosclerosis.

Angina pectoris may be mistaken for a genuine heart attack. However, the discomfort due to a heart attack usually lasts longer. In both conditions the discomfort may be intense, originating beneath the sternum (breastbone), and often radiating to the shoulder and down the arm (usually on the left side). When in doubt as to which condition is causing the discomfort, the safe procedure is to assume that the situation is the more serious of the two possibilities.

### Care and Treatment

**The person who has had previous episodes of angina pectoris has usually been instructed by his doctor to carry with him a small supply of nitroglycerine tablets. One or two of these tablets placed under the tongue at the time of an attack will cause a general relaxation of the body's arteries, which reduces the work load of the heart. This relieves the pain. In the meantime, the person is to be kept quietly at rest, lying on his back with his head and shoulders elevated slightly.**

**In addition to nitroglycerine for temporary relief, there are other drugs (such as the beta-blockers and the calcium channel antagonists) that the physician may choose to prescribe. High blood pressure, if present, should be corrected. So should anemia and so should obesity. In the cases in which the underlying cause of the angina pectoris is arteriosclerosis, the individual will do well to follow the suggestions made in the following section on coronary heart disease. This includes an appropriate program of systematic exercise within the limits of the person's tolerance. The same program which helps to prevent a coronary heart attack will benefit the person with angina pectoris.**

## CORONARY HEART DISEASE

Heart disease in its various forms stands at the top of the list of diseases that cause death and invalidism. Of the various forms of heart disease, it is coronary heart disease that largely ac-

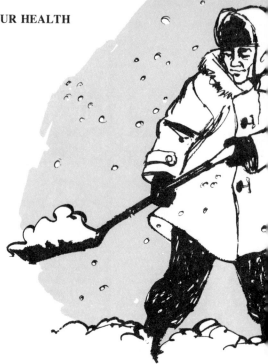

Overexertion or vigorous exercise may precipitate a heart attack.

counts for this high figure.

An average healthy man living in the United States has about one chance in five of developing coronary heart disease before he reaches 65. Notice that we mentioned the average *man*. Coronary heart disease is more common among men than among women.

It is coronary heart disease that accounts for practically all the instances of "heart attack" that strike suddenly and end, so many times, in sudden death. About 25 percent of persons who have a first heart attack die within three hours of the onset of the attack. Another 10 percent of this group of first-heart-attack victims die within the next four weeks. This leaves 65 percent who survive their first heart attack, only to live with the knowledge that they are quite vulnerable to another heart attack and that, at best, their life expectancy is reduced.

Arteriosclerosis is the basic cause of coronary heart disease. The heart is a

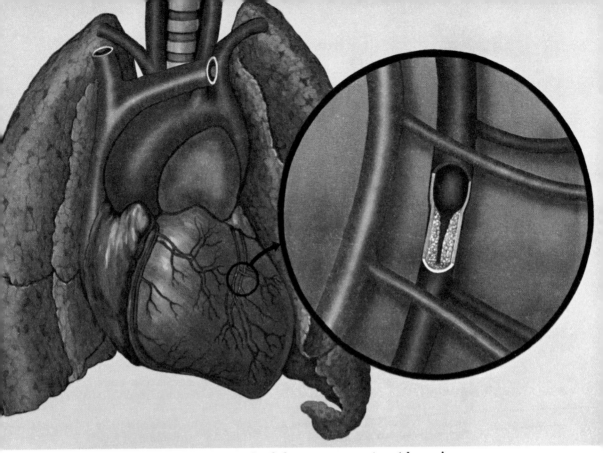

**Obstruction in a major branch of the coronary system (shown in circle), as by a coronary thrombosis, deprives a certain area of the heart wall of its blood supply, bringing on myocardial infarction.**

the chest, or even in the region of the upper part of the stomach, and often radiates to the shoulder and arm. He often feels that his chest is being squeezed. The discomfort is so intense that he experiences difficulty in breathing. He becomes weak. He may be nauseated and may vomit. He often perspires freely. His skin may be moist and cold. The skin may appear pale or dusky. He often expresses fear of impending death. The discomfort usually persists for half an hour or more.

The above description applies to the usual case of heart attack. But the symptoms may vary a great deal from case to case. Some of the associated symptoms may be absent in a particular case.

Doubt as to what is causing the symptoms, plus the natural desire to believe the best rather than the worst,

explains why so many cases of heart attack are not given the prompt care they so urgently deserve. The care the victim receives during the first few minutes of his attack may make the difference between life and death.

The American Heart Association puts it this way: "Don't you wait. If you think someone is having a heart attack, call the fire department rescue squad immediately. Seconds count. Don't wait for severe pain, dizziness, fainting, sweating, or shortness of breath. . . . Don't let the fear of embarrassment delay your call. If you're wrong about the existence of a heart attack, it doesn't matter. If you're right, nothing could matter more."

You may live near a fire department that has a rescue squad. But call whatever help is available: a doctor, an ambulance. Many ambulances are now operated by trained paramedics who can give necessary emergency care to a patient even before he is transported to the hospital emergency room.

### Care and Treatment

*Immediate Care:*

1. Call for a doctor, the fire department rescue squad, or an ambulance. Make the message urgent, stating that a person is having a heart attack. Give your name, address, and telephone number.

2. Place the victim in a half-reclining position with his head and shoulders elevated slightly. Keep him in this position until seen by the doctor or until trained help arrives.

3. Insist that the victim remain absolutely at rest, not even moving a finger.

4. Loosen the victim's clothing where it might constrict his neck or waist.

5. Allow him to breathe fresh air. If a tank of oxygen is available, play a gentle stream of oxygen over the victim's face so he can breathe it.

6. If tablets of nitroglycerine are available, place one of these under the victim's tongue, allowing it to be dissolved there.

7. When trained help arrives, follow instructions.

**Treatment for heart symptoms typically includes bed rest.**

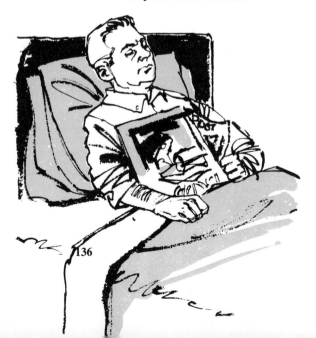

8. Allow the patient to be transferred to the emergency room of a hospital or, if available, to a hospital coronary-care unit.

*Treating the Heart Attack Patient.* The proper care for a person who has just suffered a heart attack requires professional expertise and technical skill. It is best accomplished in the coronary-care unit of a hospital. Here the necessary equipment is available for monitoring the heart's action continuously, 24 hours a day. The personnel of a coronary-care unit are trained to deal with each complication that may develop.

The principle of caring for a recent case of heart attack requires that the workload of the heart be reduced as much as possible throughout the time the damaged portion of the heart is healing. The patient must be kept at rest. Sometimes medicines are necessary to relieve pain. In some cases oxygen is administered to make the patient's breathing easier.

*Rehabilitation After Heart Attack.* At any one time, approximately 7,000,000 persons residing in the United States have had at least one heart attack. The methods of helping these persons to resume productive life programs and, at the same time, of prolonging their lives have improved through recent years.

A patient recovering from a heart attack should have a bland diet low in calories—so low that he loses some weight. As he continues to improve, the number of calories in his daily diet can be raised to about 1500, still on the low side compared with the average diet for an adult.

Such a person should live at a slower pace than customary until his heart has completely healed. If he has been a smoker, he should permanently discontinue the use of cigarettes.

The person who has had a heart attack benefits greatly thereafter by following a program of systematic phys-

# Cardiovascular Disorders; Blood Vessel Diseases

## A.  Cardiovascular Diseases

When we speak of cardiovascular disorders we refer to those conditions in which the heart and/or the blood vessels function abnormally, with the result that the circulation of blood is altered in some unfavorable way. We use the word *cardiovascular* in describing these disorders because the heart (cardio) and the blood vessels (vascular) work together as a functioning unit.

### COLD EXTREMITIES (POOR CIRCULATION)

Normal warmth in the hands and feet depends on an adequate circulation of blood through the extremities. A decrease in the flow of blood through these parts may be caused automatically by the body's need to conserve heat, by a decline in the heart's ability to pump blood, or by a reduced capacity of the blood vessels to convey blood. A reduction in blood volume to the arms and legs may be brought about by the action of the nerves as they restrict the size of the blood vessels and reduce the flow of blood, as in emotional tension or when a person is studying intently. Poor circulation of blood to the hands and feet may occur in shock, in heart disease, in advanced arteriosclerosis, in thromboangiitis obliterans (Buerger's disease), or in Reynaud's disease.

### EDEMA (SWELLING OF THE TISSUES)

Edema consists of an accumulation of excess fluid in certain of the body's tissues. The extra fluid accumulates outside of the capillaries in the spaces between the cells. Thus the tissues become soggy and swollen.

Normally, a continual exchange of fluid takes place between the blood within the capillaries and the tissue spaces outside the capillaries. The walls of the capillaries permit water and relatively small molecules of other substances to pass through. Larger protein molecules and blood cells do not normally penetrate the capillary wall. A certain amount of fluid in the tissue spaces enters the lymph vessels instead of reentering the blood capillaries.

Four factors control the balance of fluid which enters and leaves the capillaries: (1) The osmotic pressure of the blood plasma as compared with that of the tissue fluid. This pressure depends in large part upon the presence of protein molecules (primarily albumin) in the blood plasma. The higher osmotic pressure of the plasma retards the escape of fluid from the capillaries. (2) The height of blood pressure within the capillaries. High blood pressure within the capillaries favors the escape of fluid from the capillaries. (3) The condition of the capillary walls. Only an abnormal capillary wall permits the escape of protein molecules. (4) The capacity of the lymph vessels to carry fluid. When these are obstructed, the fluid which would normally follow this route tends to accumulate in the tissue spaces.

1. *Edema in Heart Disease.* When the heart fails to put out as much blood as the body's tissues require, the kidneys respond by decreasing the volume of fluid they excrete. This increases the volume of total body fluid, with a resulting rise of blood pressure within the capillaries. Then, as mentioned in item number two of the preceding paragraph, edema occurs. The edema (swelling of tissues) is noticed first in the ankles of ambulatory patients and in the sacral region of bed patients. The edema is typically more severe at the end of the day.

2. *Edema in Kidney Disease.* Certain forms of kidney disease allow the escape of albumin from the blood plasma into the urine. Albumin is thus lost from the body faster than it can be replenished. The consequent lowering of the blood's osmotic pressure permits an excess of fluid to escape through the capillary walls into the tissue spaces.

3. *Edema in Cirrhosis of the Liver.* In cirrhosis the liver's production of protein declines, with a consequent lowering of the blood's osmotic pressure. This favors the development of edema. Also, cirrhosis hinders the flow of blood coming to the liver from other abdominal organs and this causes an increase of blood pressure in the capillaries of these organs. This results in an accumulation of fluid in the abdominal cavity (ascites).

4. *Edema in Malnutrition.* Here, the edema is attributed to damage to the capillary wall and to a reduced intake of protein materials from which the albumin of the blood plasma is normally derived.

5. *Edema in Local Inflammation.* Blood tends to stagnate in an inflamed tissue area. The capillary walls are damaged and local swelling occurs.

6. *Edema in Allergy.* The tissue swelling which occurs in various allergic manifestations (hives, hay fever, angioneurotic edema, etc.) is attributed to the effect of histamine (a chemical liberated in the allergic reaction) on the walls of the capillaries.

7. *Edema in Local Injury.* Local injury, whether by mechanical force, heat, or cold, causes damage to the capillaries, with resulting local swelling.

8. *Edema in Poisoning and Toxemia.* Poisonous substances containing arsenic, lead, antimony, gold, or mercury, as well as the toxins produced in such diseases as diphtheria and scarlet fever, damage the capillaries and thus permit the escape of excess fluid into the tissues.

9. *Edema From Obstruction of the Veins.* When the return of blood through a vein is impeded, the consequent increase of blood pressure within the capillaries results in a swelling of all tissues drained by this particular vein. In some cases tumors compress the large veins which enter the heart, and the resulting edema may involve large portions of the body.

10. *Edema From Obstruction of the Lymph Vessels.* The lymph vessels may be obstructed when involved in a region of inflammation, when invaded

unnecessary conversation.

5. Administer drinking water cautiously. If the patient is conscious and vomiting, it is wise to offer him small drinks of water to make up in part for the loss of his body fluids. Give this a sip at a time. Use no alcoholic drinks.

6. Transport the victim carefully. Keep him in a reclining position while being transported and avoid all excitement and unnecessary changes in position.

## HIGH BLOOD PRESSURE (HYPERTENSION)

High blood pressure is a common disorder, occurring during the lifetime of one out of five Americans. It is not a disease in the sense of being caused by germs or resulting from deterioration of certain of the body's tissues. Rather, it represents the body's response to conditions that trigger a constriction of blood vessels throughout the body and thus increase the heart's work load.

We take high blood pressure so seriously because it sets the stage for certain life-threatening complications such as stroke, heart disease, and kidney failure.

Quite arbitrarily doctors consider blood pressure greater than 160/90 within the range of high blood pressure. To understand these figures we must first consider how blood pressure is measured—the meaning of these two readings, the high and the low. See chapter 7 in this volume.

Average normal blood pressures are lower in children (90/60 at age 6) than in young adults (120/80). The normal range for blood pressure in a healthy young adult is 90 to 140 for the systolic and 60 to 90 for the diastolic. The blood pressure tends to increase slightly as a person becomes older, even though he is in perfectly normal health. Persistent readings above 160 systolic or above 90 diastolic fall into the range of high blood pressure. Notice that we said *persistent* readings above these figures. A single blood pressure reading may not indicate truly a person's actual level of blood pressure. Momentary ex-

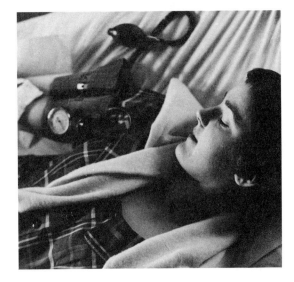

citement or nervousness may shoot the pressure up higher than ordinary. In fact, the temporary elevation of blood pressures is one of the body's normal reactions to stress, excitement, or any emergency. Therefore, a series of at least three blood pressure readings should be taken at different times when the individual is at rest in order to determine his real, average blood pressure.

Many factors may cause a person's blood pressure to remain high, any one of which or any combination of which may be to blame in a given case. Overeating with resultant obesity is a common causative factor. The use of large amounts of salt in the food is a contributing factor, as indicated by the observation that in countries where persons use relatively little salt the incidence of high blood pressure is low. Stress—physical, social, and business—is a factor in producing high blood pressure. The smoking of a single cigarette may temporarily raise the systolic blood pressure between 5 and 10 points. Persistent smoking is a contributing factor to the development of high blood pressure.

Acute infections, such as tonsillitis, sometimes lead to kidney disease, which may bring with it high blood pressure. In some cases the increased pressure is a natural compensatory mechanism to maintain a normal filtration rate through the hardened walls of the small blood vessels in the kidneys. Kidney disease of the slowly progressive type is often accompanied by hardening of the arteries, high blood pressure, and enlargement of the heart. Sudden attacks of convulsions in pregnant women (eclampsia) and other kidney disorders of pregnancy are associated with an increase in blood pressure.

Many cases of high blood pressure are accompanied by practically no telltale symptoms. In fact, blood pressure has been described as the "silent killer." It is therefore wise to make sure that your blood pressure is measured each time you visit the doctor's office.

High blood pressure is typically associated with the development of arteriosclerosis (hardening of the arteries). Therefore the same precautions that a person takes to retard the development of arteriosclerosis are also effective in delaying or preventing the development of high blood pressure. The ideal way of life centers around the maintenance of fitness as described in chapter 52, volume 1.

### Care and Treatment

**As already stated, the hazard of high blood pressure consists of the risk of life-threatening complications, including stroke, heart disease, and kidney failure. It has been clearly demonstrated that the risk of these complications, even in a person who already has high blood pressure, is greatly reduced when the person follows a care and treatment program that brings his blood pressure into the normal range.**

**1. First attention should be given to eliminating the conditions that may have contributed to the high blood**

**Therapy for high blood pressure includes abundant fruit in the diet.**

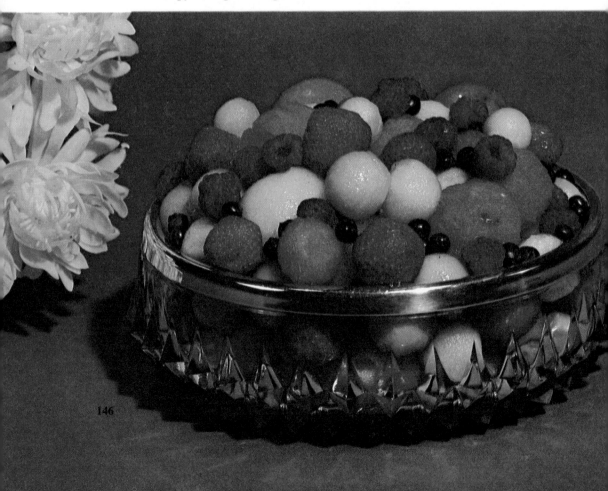

146

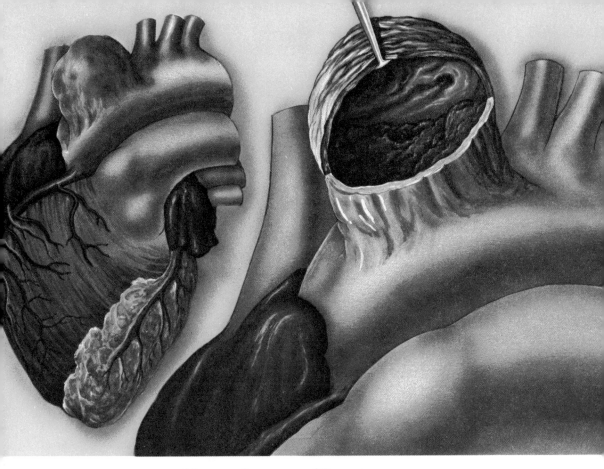

**Diagram of aneurysm of the aorta.**

bly a pulsating bulging of the chest wall.

An aneurysm located in the descending portion of the thoracic aorta may produce no symptoms. However, if large enough to press on one or more of the ribs or on the spinal column, such an aneurysm may cause degeneration of bone accompanied by pain. An aneurysm in the abdominal portion of the aorta is typically indicated by a pulsating mass deep in the central part of the abdomen. There may be pain in the upper abdomen, lower back, or groin.

Aneurysms or arteries within the skull are likely to cause headache, especially on exertion. They also frequently hinder the normal action of some of the cranial nerves, giving rise to signs and symptoms that help the physician to determine what is wrong. Rupture of and bleeding from an aneurysm within the skull is one of the conditions that can cause a stroke.

### Care and Treatment

The preferred method of treatment of aneurysms is by surgical repair. Surgical operations for this condition are delicate and hazardous and require the skill of a surgeon trained in vascular surgery or in neurosurgery (for those aneurysms located inside the skull). For patients with aneurysm whose physical condition would not tolerate surgery, rupture of the aneurysm may be delayed or possibly prevented by a program of reducing the blood pressure by means of medications designed for this purpose. Even for those cases of aneurysm treated by surgery, the mortality rate is about 30 percent.

### STROKE

A stroke is caused by damage to some part of the brain because of an interruption of the blood supply to this part. The exact symptoms of a particular case depend on the particular part of the brain affected, on the size of the brain area deprived of its blood supply, and on whether the deprivation of blood to this part is temporary (as in a transient ischemic attack) or is permanent.

The demands of the brain for a continuous supply of fresh blood are so great that one fifth of the blood pumped by the heart is delivered to the brain. A complete interruption of blood supply to any part of the brain causes permanent damage to the brain cells within about five minutes.

About 80 percent of the deaths from stroke occur in people 65 years old or above. Four out of five persons survive their first attack of stroke, but these are often handicapped to a greater or lesser degree, perhaps by a paralysis of some muscles.

Although the onset of a stroke is sudden, the underlying disease condition is usually of long standing. Stroke may be caused by the formation of a blood clot (thrombus) inside of one of the vessels that supplies the brain—a complication of arteriosclerosis. Stroke may be caused by the lodgment of a floating fragment of blood clot (embolus) in one of the arteries of the brain. Or it may be caused by a rupture of the wall of an artery in the brain, with consequent escape of blood into the brain tissue. Such rupture may be brought about by high blood pressure forcing blood through a weakened vessel wall, as in arteriosclerosis or in aneurysm of the involved vessel.

For a more complete discussion of stroke, including symptoms and long-range plan of treatment, see chapter 4, volume 3. For instruction on the first-aid treatment of a person who has just suffered a stroke, see chapter 23, volume 3.

## BUERGER'S DISEASE
## THROMBOANGIITIS OBLITERANS)

In Buerger's disease there develops an inflammation of the lining of blood vessels in the extremities. The arteries

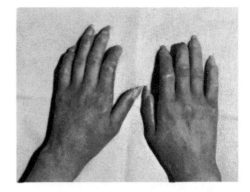

**Buerger's disease affects the hands and feet, often causing ulceration.**

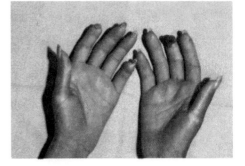

are more commonly affected than the veins, and the legs are involved more commonly than the arms. The inflammation involves a partial or complete closure of the lumen of the affected vessel. The symptoms, therefore, are caused by a marked reduction or even a loss of blood supply to the part of the body ordinarily supplied by this vessel. Buerger's disease occurs most frequently in men aged 20 to 40 and, most often, in those who smoke.

Although all four extremities may be affected, usually only one leg is most severely involved. This extremity is colder than normal, painful, tender, and often of a mottled red appearance. Little or no pulse can be felt in it. In severe cases ulcers and even gangrene develop in the limb now deprived of its blood supply.

Exercise intensifies the pain of Buerger's disease, but "rest pain" may occur in severe cases, especially at night.

The exact cause of Buerger's disease is not known, but there appears to be an hereditary factor. Also, the use of cigarettes seems to predispose to this illness.

### Care and Treatment

**The person with Buerger's disease should avoid exercise which causes pain and should protect himself against cold or mechanical injury to the affected part. The involved extremity should be kept scrupulously clean and dry in the hope of avoiding ulceration.**

**It is very important that cigarette smoking be avoided.**

**In severe cases, it is best for the patient to remain in bed with the affected limb slightly lowered so as to encourage the circulation of blood in the affected part. Circulation in the affected limb can be somewhat improved by applying heat to the corresponding unaffected limb, as by suspending a light bulb at a safe distance in an overlying, tunnel-shaped framework (electric light cradle).**

**A physician should be retained to supervise the continuing care of a patient with Buerger's disease. In those cases in which gangrene develops as a complication, amputation of the affected limb may become necessary.**

## RAYNAUD'S DISEASE

Raynaud's disease is another illness, as in Buerger's disease, in which the blood supply to distant parts of the body is reduced. The fundamental difference between the two is that in Raynaud's disease the reduction of blood flow is the result of nervous stimulation through the autonomic nerves which causes the delicate muscle fibers in the walls of small arteries to contract, thus reducing the caliber of these arteries. Raynaud's disease affects the hands more commonly than the feet. It occurs more frequently in women than in men. The illness occurs typically in attacks accompanied by numbness, tingling, pain, and blanching. Aggravating factors include emotional upset, expo-

sure to cold, and the intake of nicotine as in any form of tobacco. In severe cases the skin and subcutaneous tissues of the fingers become dry and shrunken. In occasional cases, gangrenous spots develop. In the usual attack the discomfort may last for minutes or even for a few hours.

### Care and Treatment

**The discomfort of an attack of Raynaud's disease may be somewhat relieved by immersing the affected member or members in warm (not hot) water.**

**The long-range relief of the symptoms of Raynaud's disease depends upon removing or avoiding the aggravating conditions. A person with this tendency should avoid exposure to cold, should avoid nervous or emotional strain, and should avoid activities that previous experience has proved may precipitate an attack. The use of tobacco in any form should be avoided.**

## BLEEDING (HEMORRHAGE)

Bleeding may occur as part of the process of disease in various organs of the body, as mentioned in chapter 6, this volume. It may occur as a result of damage to arteries, capillaries, or veins. It may occur in connection with one of the bleeding disorders mentioned in the next chapter. In some cases of injury and in some cases of disease, bleeding may be so profuse as to threaten life within a matter of minutes. The first-aid handling of serious bleeding is considered in chapter 23, volume 3.

## VARICOSE VEINS

Varicose veins are veins which become swollen and tortuous because of the increased volume and pressure of the blood they contain. The usual usage of the term applies to conspicuous, unsightly veins appearing just under the skin of the leg.

An estimated 10 percent of all adults have conspicuous varicose veins. The problem occurs twice as commonly

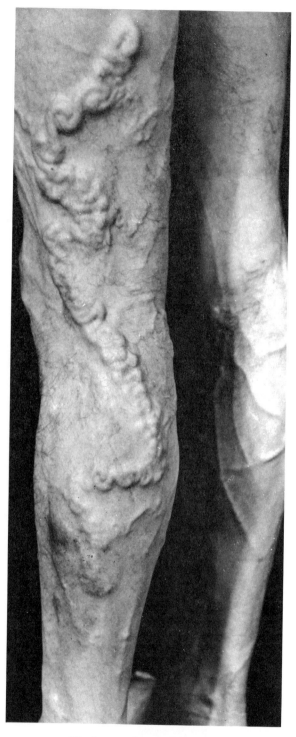

Varicose veins as they appear in the thigh and below the knee.

among women as among men. The fundamental cause is a stretching of the vein by way of a partial stagnation of the blood which the vein conveys, with the result that the valves within the vein which should prevent the backward flow of blood now become incompetent.

Most varicose veins develop in persons under 40 and tend to persist thereafter. Some people are more susceptible, supposedly because of an inherited factor of tissue weakness. In women, pregnancy and pelvic tumors predispose to the condition. The wearing of tight bands or garters about the legs is an aggravating cause. Occupations that require long hours of standing cause varicose veins in many people. Aching in the leg, swelling, eczema of the skin, and varicose ulcers may occur as complications of varicose veins.

The development of varicose ulcers is a serious complication. The wearing of support hose in a case of varicose veins may prevent the development of ulcers. When ulcers develop, they are usually located just above the ankle. They are hard to heal and may recur after healing.

Internal varicose veins may occur in the rectum or occasionally in the esophagus near where it enters the stomach. Rectal varicose veins are commonly called hemorrhoids. They are readily detectable, and surgery is the effective cure. The varicose veins in the lower end of the esophagus are neither easy to detect nor easy to treat. Their presence is usually not known until they rupture, causing a serious hemorrhage. They commonly form as a complication of cirrhosis of the liver.

### Care and Treatment

For cases of moderately severe varicose veins, some commonsense procedures may keep the condition from becoming worse and may, hopefully, avoid the development of varicose ulcers: (1) avoid stationary standing for long periods of time; (2) change the position of the legs every few minutes so that the use of the leg

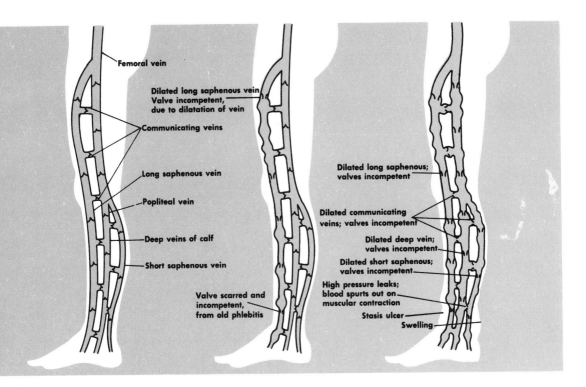

Femoral vein

Dilated long saphenous vein
Valve incompetent,
due to dilatation of vein

Communicating veins

Long saphenous vein

Popliteal vein

Deep veins of calf

Short saphenous vein

Valve scarred and
incompetent,
from old phlebitis

Dilated long saphenous;
valves incompetent

Dilated communicating
veins; valves incompetent

Dilated deep vein;
valves incompetent

Dilated short saphenous;
valves incompetent

High pressure leaks;
blood spurts out on
muscular contraction

Stasis ulcer

Swelling

Varicose veins develop when valves permitting normal blood flow
(1) become incompetent and allow blood flow to become retrograde
(2), resulting in chronic venous insufficiency (3).

muscles will compress the enlarged veins and move the blood on its way; (3) lie down and elevate the legs to a level above that of the heart for a few minutes several times a day; (4) wear elastic stockings to compress the veins and keep the blood from stagnating within them.

If swelling, eczema of the skin, or varicose ulcers are present, use alternate hot and cold foot and leg baths for 20 minutes twice a day. Begin with two minutes in the hot and half a minute in the cold, and gradually increase the time of the cold until it is also two minutes. After each treatment, it is essential to dry the skin gently but thoroughly.

For varicose ulcers, apply a mild antiseptic ointment and cover with a sterile but firm-fitting bandage.

For troublesome cases and especially for those in which ulcers develop, consult a physician. Surgical removal of varicose veins is still the most satisfactory treatment for the difficult cases.

## PHLEBITIS AND THROMBOPHLEBITIS

Phlebitis is a condition in which a vein, particularly its lining layer, becomes inflamed. Usually, in the course of the inflammation, blood platelets adhere to the inflamed lining of the vein and a blood clot forms within the vein. The blood clot often completely obstructs the vein. This constitutes thrombophlebitis. There then develops the possibility that a portion of the blood clot may break away and move along the course of the vein until it lodges in some other part of the body. This serious complication (embolism) is discussed in the item which follows.

Thrombophlebitis occurs most commonly in the veins of the thigh and leg.

155

# *Blood Diseases*\*

Blood is composed of cells and plasma. See the discussion of blood in chapter 7, this volume. Plasma is largely water in which are dissolved minerals, proteins, gases, and other chemicals that assist in the work done by the blood. Whether all are in the right proportions or not depends on the state of nutrition and metabolism of the body and to a lesser extent on the activity of the blood-forming organs. Most commonly, plasma abnormalities occur when something goes wrong with the respiratory, digestive, or excretory organs. Discussion of such problems in this chapter will be limited, however, to conditions which affect the protein of the plasma and thus directly alter blood clotting.

Blood cells are produced in special tissues or organs. Bone marrow, the largest blood-forming organ, supplies red cells, certain white cells called granulocytes, and platelets. Other white cells (the lymphocytes and plasma cells) are formed in the spleen, lymph nodes, and other lymphoid tissues. Granulocytes once were considered the most important of the white cells because their activity could be easily observed in the laboratory. Recently, however, it has been discovered that lymphocytes and plasma cells are very important in overcoming infections caused by viruses and in maintaining immunity against certain diseases; *e.g.,* measles, whooping cough, and smallpox.

Diseases of the blood may involve red cells, white cells, platelets, or plasma constituents. The effects of disease may result in too few or too many of the item concerned. When there are too many red cells, the condition is called polycythemia; when there are too few red cells, we speak of anemia. An increased number of white cells occurs in response to an infection or in a case of leukemia and is called leukocytosis. A decrease in white cells is called leukopenia. A condition in which there are too few platelets is known as thrombocytopenia. Conditions in which there is an excess of plasma protein are rare, but too little of the right kind of protein in the plasma may cause abnormal bleeding problems, as in hemophilia. Too little of the gamma globulin component of the plasma's protein causes a striking susceptibility to infection.

In the present chapter discussion of the characteristics, causes, and treatments of blood diseases are necessarily

\*The authors and publishers acknowledge the significant contribution to the content of this chapter by Irvin N. Kuhn, M.D., Professor of Internal Medicine, and Jeffrey D. Cao, M.D., Assistant Professor of Pathology, both of Loma Linda University School of Medicine.

# Disorders of the Skeletal Structures

In this chapter we consider problems and diseases relating to the bones, the tendons and ligaments, and the joints. The collagen vascular diseases are considered here because they involve the connective tissues which are a part of the body's supporting system. Amputations and their related problems are also considered.

## A. Involvements of Bones and Skeletal Parts

### FRACTURES

A bone fracture consists of a break in bone structure. A fracture may be caused by a fall, by a sudden impact (as in an automobile accident), or by a crushing injury.

A child's bone, containing less calcium and phosphorus than an adult's, often cracks and bends without breaking completely. This is a so-called greenstick fracture. The common type of fracture of an adult bone is called a closed fracture. The break is typically across the shaft of a long bone with no broken ends protruding. A more serious type of fracture, in which the ends of the broken bone pierce the muscles and skin, is called an open fracture.

When doubt exists on whether a bone has been fractured, the patient should be handled as though there is a broken bone. Usually, however, the first-aider can make a good guess by remembering the usual indications of a fracture: (1) the injured person has felt a sudden "snap" in the involved part of his body; (2) the site of a fracture is tender to the touch and painful; (3) swelling usually develops at the site of a fracture; (4) the injured part may be out of shape; (5) the victim guards the injured part of his body, avoiding any attempt to use it; (6) moving the injured part may produce a very uncomfortable grating of bone; and (7) an injured limb may appear shorter than the opposite limb.

### Care and Treatment

**The first-aid care of a person with a fractured bone is given in chapter 23, volume 3.**

### CLUBFOOT

The usual type of clubfoot with which an infant is born involves a congenital abnormality of the bone that acts as the "spool" of the ankle joint. When such a foot is allowed to continue untreated, a crippling deformity persists.

# Types of fractures

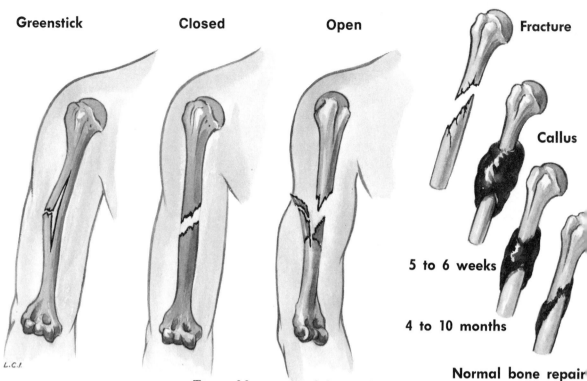

**Greenstick**     **Closed**     **Open**     Fracture

Callus

5 to 6 weeks

4 to 10 months

**Normal bone repair**

L.C.L.

Types of fractures and the repair of bone.

### Care and Treatment

Professional care should be arranged. In most cases, a manipulation of the baby's foot into normal position with casts to hold it in this position for a few weeks or months will help it to develop normally. Appropriate bracing and corrective shoes may be used for a while during early childhood. In the more serious cases, surgical correction may be necessary.

## BOWLEGS AND KNOCK-KNEES

Bowing of the legs is normal in a newborn baby, and this condition persists for a few months. Normally the legs become straighter as the child develops. Bowlegs in a young child should not be considered a deformity unless and until the normal straightening is much delayed.

A child's legs are not likely to become permanently bowed from early walking if his diet contains adequate bone-building materials. Many children have walked at an age as young as nine months and younger without prolonging or increasing the bowing of their legs.

A knock-kneed baby is a rarity, but in a growing child the change from early bowing may sometimes continue until knock-knees develop. This is more often true of girls than of boys.

Rarely bowlegs or knock-knees are secondary to disorders of the growing centers of the bones at the knee or to such diseases as rickets, scurvy, or cerebral palsy. Overweight may be a causative factor. The habit of sitting on the floor with the knees flexed and the feet and legs to the outside of the thighs may lead to knock-knees and "pigeon toes."

### Care and Treatment

If babies are given enough milk and foods containing an abundance of vitamins C and D and are not urged to walk before they do so on their own, bowlegs and knock-knees will not likely develop.

If, in spite of good care, bowlegs are not improving by the end of a

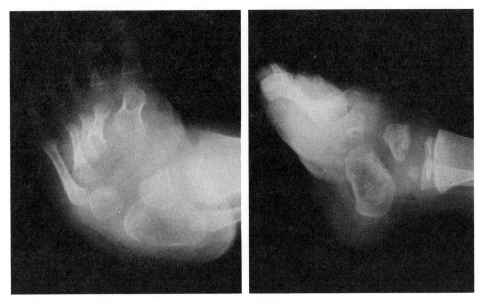

X rays of clubfoot.

child's first year, a physician should be consulted. He may advise the use of braces and/or modification of the shoes to change the direction of the weight-bearing thrust.

## RICKETS AND OSTEOMALACIA

Both rickets and osteomalacia are caused by a deficiency of vitamin D. Rickets occurs during childhood and osteomalacia during adulthood. In each case a misshaping of the bones of the body occurs. For further details, see chapter 17, volume 1, for a discussion of rickets, and chapter 12, volume 3, for a discussion of osteomalacia.

## CURVATURE OF THE SPINE

Spine curvature in which the hump is toward the back is called hunchback or kyphosis and that with the hollow in the back is called swayback or lordosis. When the curvature is side to side, it is called scoliosis. Some cases of curvature may be caused by long-continued faulty posture. Hereditary faults in the development of the bones, diseases of the vertebrae, or a weakness of certain muscles are possible causes of spinal curvature. Once a curvature becomes established, particularly in childhood,

the curve increases progressively during the growth period and may eventually result in serious problems with breathing.

### Care and Treatment

Parents and teachers should be alert to notice children in whom a spinal curvature of any type is beginning. Such curvature may start as early as age 10 or 12 years. When such is observed, professional care should be arranged. It is important that children in school be provided with seats and desks of proper height and adjustment so as to favor a normal sitting position.

When a noticeable curvature develops, a physician who specializes in orthopedics should be consulted. Plaster casts, braces, special exercises, and even surgery may be needed to correct the condition.

## OSTEOMYELITIS

Osteomyelitis consists of an infection and partial destruction of some particular bone. It may be caused by various germs but most commonly by the staphylococcus.

In osteomyelitis that occurs in the

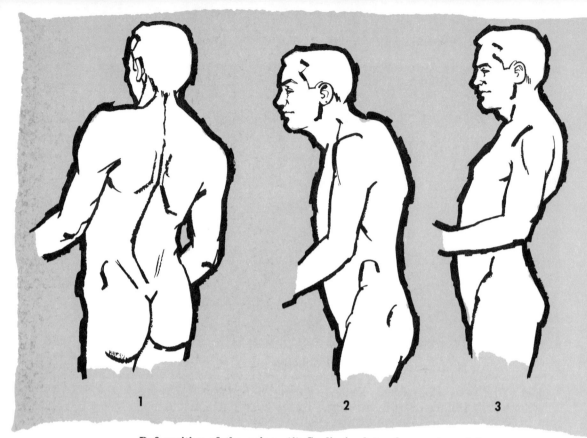

Deformities of the spine: (1) Scoliosis, lateral curvature (observe the lowering of the right shoulder); (2) kyphosis (hunchback); (3) lordosis (note how curvature forms a hollow).

younger age group (most commonly between ages 10 and 15) the germs usually come from an infection in some distant part of the body, such as from a boil, from an infection of the middle ear, or from pneumonia. The germs are carried by the blood and lodge in the marrow of a bone, where they cause a progressing destruction of bone tissue.

In typical adult osteomyelitis, the germs are more often placed in or near the bone at the time of injury.

The symptoms of osteomyelitis include acute pain in the affected bone when that part of the body is moved. Also evidences of infection such as chills and fever appear.

### Care and Treatment

**Osteomyelitis is a serious condition, and the care of the case must be under the supervision of a physician. It is best treated by the precise and vigorous use of the proper antibiotic medication, with the patient in the hospital. The choice of the antibiotic depends on the kind of infection present. Medication must be continued for several weeks. In cases in which the infection has made considerable progress, it may be necessary for the surgeon to remove fragments of devitalized bone.**

### BACK PAIN AND BACKACHE

Discomfort in the back, in its various forms, is one of the most common symptoms.

Obesity is a common cause of backache. It causes poor posture, with resulting strain and fatigue of the structures in the back. Back pain is often referred from problems in the pelvic organs. Thus it may occur during menstruation, in pregnancy, and in inflammation of the pelvic organs. It commonly occurs in kidney disease. Pain in the back may be an early symptom of a generalized infection. It may result from an injury.

For a further consideration of back pain and backache, see chapter 7, volume 3.

## HERNIATED DISK INVOLVEMENT (SLIPPED DISK; HERNIATED DISK; RUPTURED DISK)

The vertebral column (spinal column) is the mainstay of the skeleton. It is subject to tremendous mechanical forces, as in lifting, jumping, twisting, and carrying heavy weights. Between each vertebra and its neighbor there is interposed a cushionlike disk of fibrocartilage (an intervertebral disk). It is these disks, by way of their resiliency, that permit the bending and twisting movements of which the vertebral column is capable. Each intervertebral disk is composed of an elastic central part, called the nucleus pulposus, and a surrounding ring of dense tissue, designated as the annulus fibrosus.

Between the bony processes of each vertebra and its neighbor there emerges a pair of spinal nerves—nerves leading from the spinal cord to some particular part of the body or the extremities.

Injuries to the intervertebral disks constitute the most common type of vertebral column injury. Such injury may be caused by heavy lifting, by a fall, by an automobile accident, by striking the head while diving, or, very commonly, by elusive, recurring forces of pressure that cause the disks to deteriorate. Immediately following an injury that damages an intervertebral disk, the patient will usually suffer pain for a few days, experiencing a "catch in the back" or a "crick in the neck." This discomfort is caused by torn ligaments or strained muscles. It may be some time later, possibly after several incidents of discomfort, that the nucleus pulposus at the center of the intervertebral disk actually squeezes through a damaged or weak part of the annulus fibrosus and brings pressure against an adjacent nerve root. This pressure causes severe pain and possible weakness of the muscles supplied

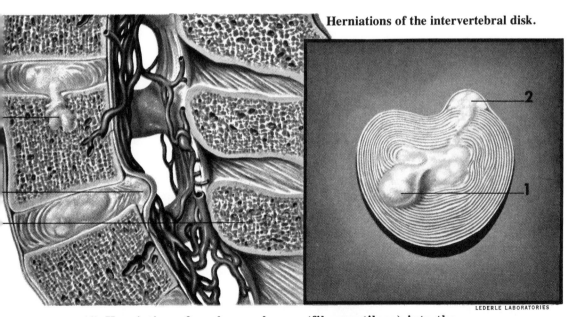

**Herniations of the intervertebral disk.**

LEDERLE LABORATORIES

**(1) Herniation of nucleus pulposus (fibrocartilage) into the spongiosa of the vertebra. (2) Herniation of nucleus pulposus beneath the posterior longitudinal ligament. (3) Spinous process.**

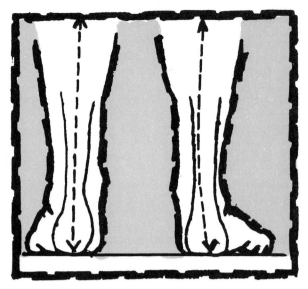

One manifestation of flatfoot is an outward deviation, shown on right, as compared with a normal foot, shown on left.

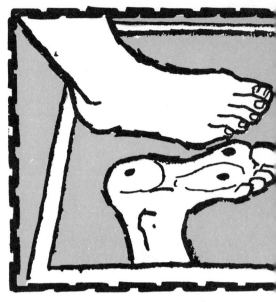

Normal distribution of body weight on the foot, the points bearing the major portion reflected in mirror.

Footprints on wet floor: A, of a normal foot; B, C, and D, of increasing degrees of flatfoot.

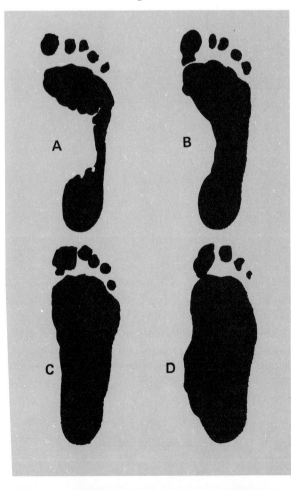

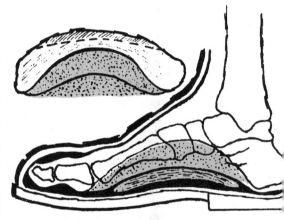

Diagram showing how arch support in a shoe helps a patient suffering from flatfoot.

or by long-continued strain on the ligaments. If a person whose leg and foot muscles are weak from too little use suddenly begins to exercise vigorously, the muscles cannot support the arches of his feet. This failure throws an added burden on the ligaments, which then stretch, causing the pain. The same result may come from a rapid increase in body weight. It may be caused by an

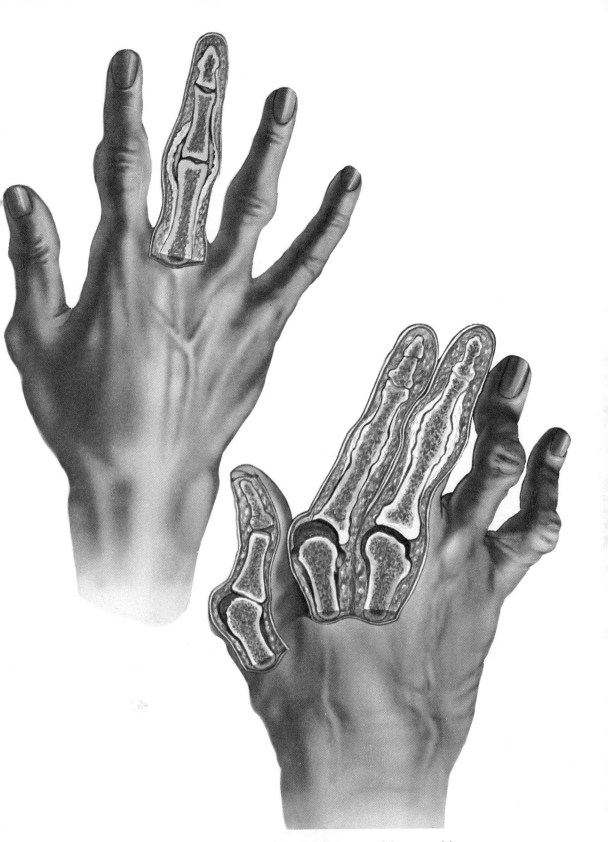

**Rheumatoid arthritis. Note swelling of joints caused by synovitis and effusion. Right: Advanced case, showing deformity from stiffness and partial dislocation of joints.**

tient avoid straining the joints presently involved and also that he reduce his general activities so as to conserve his quota of vitality.

2. *Psychological Adjustment.* The patient should be provided with a fund of information regarding his disease so that he knows what to expect. He should receive encouragement to become reconciled to the handicaps which his disease produces. On the positive side, he should plan his future so that he can be productive and can experience the rewards of success. Appropriate literature may be obtained from The Arthritis Foundation, 475 Riverside Drive, New York, NY 10027.

3. *Relief of Pain.* This is accomplished, in part, by the use of dry heat to the affected parts of the body and otherwise by pain-relieving medicines, as recommended by the doctor. The commonly used medicines are the salicylates, of which aspirin is the most popular and the least harmful. The use of pain-relieving medicine introduces the danger of anemia, for these medicines may have a damaging effect on the blood-forming tissues of the body.

4. *Measures to Combat Anemia.*

Modern methods of treatment enable many arthritic patients to carry on normal activities and live useful lives.

D. TANK

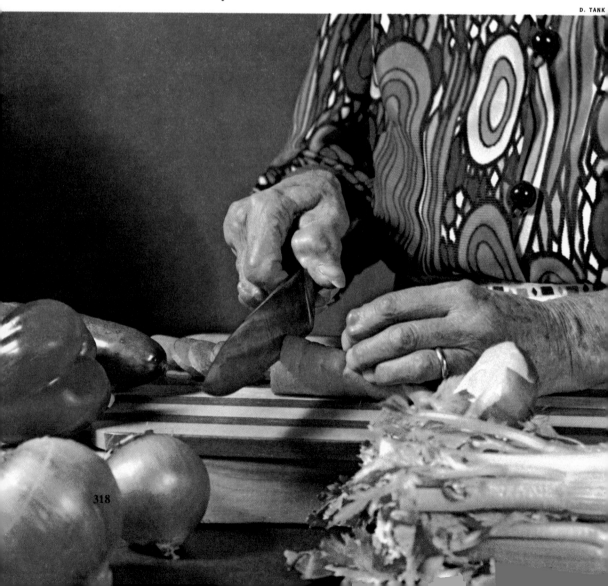

# Muscles: Their Structure, Function, and Diseases

Our modern concepts of power make us think of wheels, gears, pulleys, and belts. The human body has none of these. But it is capable of doing a great deal of work, even so.

The power of the human body is derived from its muscles. These do the work of engines in that they convert the latent energy contained in fuel into mechanical energy and heat. Muscles of just the right size to meet the needs are located throughout the body in or near the various places where power is required.

The fuel from which muscles ultimately derive their energy is the blood sugar (glucose)—along with a certain amount of fat and protein—all carried by the blood and distributed to every part of the body. In order that blood sugar may contribute energy, it must be combined with oxygen, very much as fuel in an engine must be mixed with air in order to produce power. Oxygen, as well as blood sugar, is conveyed by the blood.

## A. Structure and Function of Muscles

There are three kinds of muscle. The muscles that do the body's heavy work are called skeletal muscles, for the most part those that move the bones of the skeleton. They provide the power to straighten the back, to walk, to perform skilled movements with the hands, to breathe and talk, to turn the head from side to side, and to make the movements of facial expression.

A special kind of muscle, found in the walls of the heart, is called heart muscle. The heart performs its work day after day as long as a person lives. It rests for fraction-second periods after each heartbeat. It beats about 100,000 times a day, and its rest periods, all totaled, add up to more than 12 hours out of each 24.

The third kind of muscle is called smooth muscle or visceral muscle. It is found in the walls of blood vessels, in

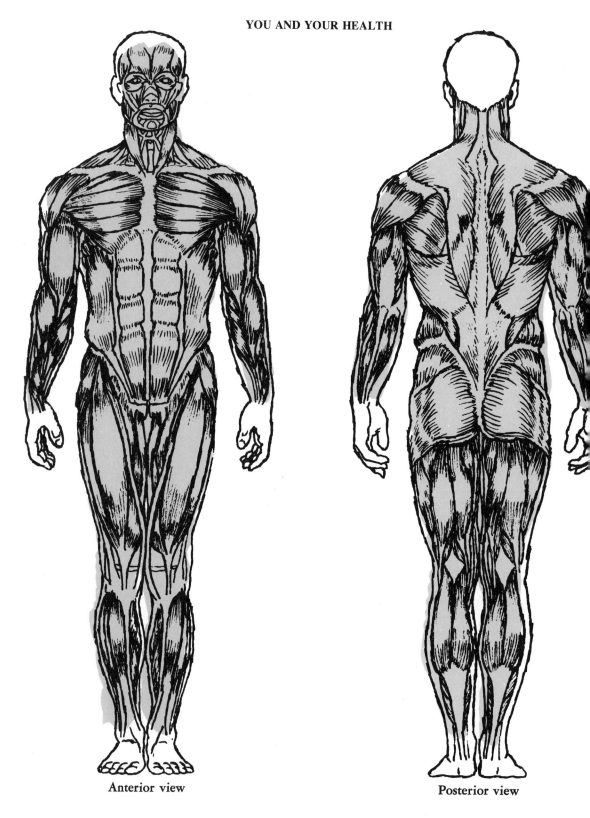

Anterior view

Posterior view

The muscles of the human body.

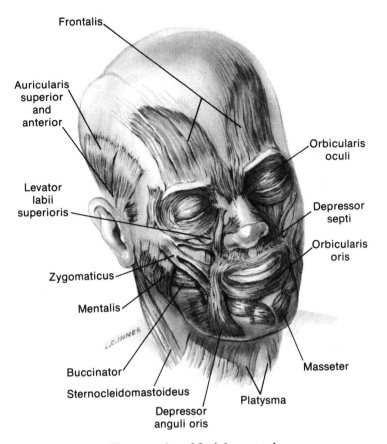

**The muscles of facial expression.**

fully, depending on the need of the moment. You use the same muscles to lift a ten-pound package of flour as to lift a piece of paper. In the latter case the muscles simply exert less power.

As explained previously, a muscle consists of many muscle fibers, and, in the case of skeletal muscle, each of these fibers is caused to contract by a tiny nerve branch. The nerves that control skeletal muscles originate either in the brain or in the spinal cord. It is here that the bodies of the nerve cells are located. Extending from the brain or spinal cord to the skeletal muscles are many nerve fibers, one fiber for each nerve cell body. As one of these nerve fibers approaches the muscle that it serves, the fiber divides into branches—sometimes only eight or ten but in other cases as many as 200.

Thus, one nerve cell in the brain or spinal cord controls as many muscle fibers as the nerve fiber has branches.

In the case of the muscles which move the eyes, the nerve fibers have about eight branches, which means that one nerve cell has only eight muscle fibers to control. This specialization explains a person's precise control over the movements of his eyes. In the case of the large muscles in one's back, however, the fiber from one nerve cell may have as many as 180 branches. Here precise control over the muscle fibers is not necessary, only approximate regulation.

The muscle fibers controlled by a single nerve cell are called a motor unit. When a particular nerve cell sends out a contraction impulse, only the muscle fibers of its motor unit respond.

331

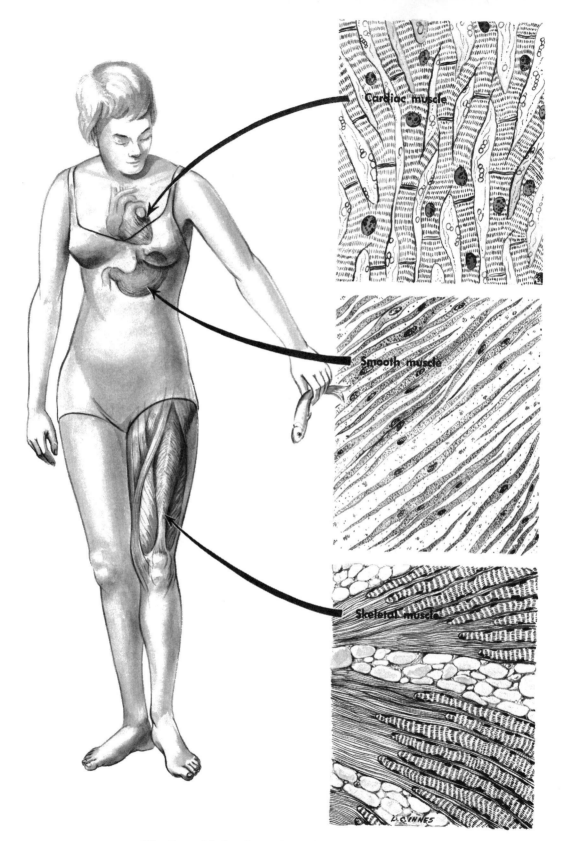

The three kinds of muscle and typical locations
where found in body.

tein can be converted into energy. But when the amount of glucose and fatty acids in the circulating blood is greater than the body's present needs require, these excess nutrients can be converted into fat, which is then stored in the fatty tissues throughout the body. Then, when a person fasts for a few hours or even for a few days, the fat stored throughout his body becomes the source of fuel.

## C. Body Heat

The chemical processes by which the molecules of food constituents are broken down into smaller molecules also produce heat. This is the source of the heat that keeps the body warm. The most active cells produce the most heat.

Muscles make up about half of the body's mass, so it is not surprising that even during rest they produce about 25 percent of the body's heat. When very active, muscles may produce up to 50 times as much heat as when at rest. The process of shivering when a person is cold is the body's automatic way of activating the muscles to produce more heat.

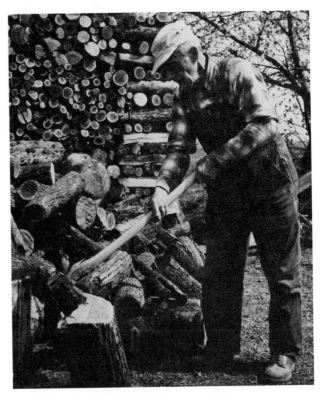

A person working hard requires more calories than a person at rest.

### Calories

It is customary when speaking of the body's energy production to measure the activities in terms of calories. A calorie is the amount of heat necessary to raise the temperature of a liter (about 1.1 quarts) of water one degree Centigrade (1.8° F.). This is the large calorie. (In certain scientific calculations not concerned with the body's energy production, the small calorie is used. A thousand small calories equal one large calorie.)

A person's energy requirements vary a great deal, of course, according to his muscular activity. An adult resting quietly in bed for 24 hours needs only 1200 to 1700 calories to provide for his body heat and to maintain the minimal activities of his tissues. This same adult, when doing long-continued, heavy work may need as much as four or five thousand calories during each 24-hour period. A person's need for calories varies also with his size and with his need for producing body heat. (The calorie requirement is greater in cold weather.)

### Metabolism

The word *metabolism* refers to the various processes of cell activity occurring throughout the body. These processes require the expenditure of the body's fuel. And the rate of fuel consumption is measured in calories. When the body's cells are exceptionally active, we say that the metabolic rate runs high. When the activity of the cells is at slow pace, we say the metabolic rate runs low. Even when a person lies quietly in bed, the activity of his cells throughout the body requires a certain minimum consumption of fuel. Although the muscles are not being used in exercise, the body's metabo-

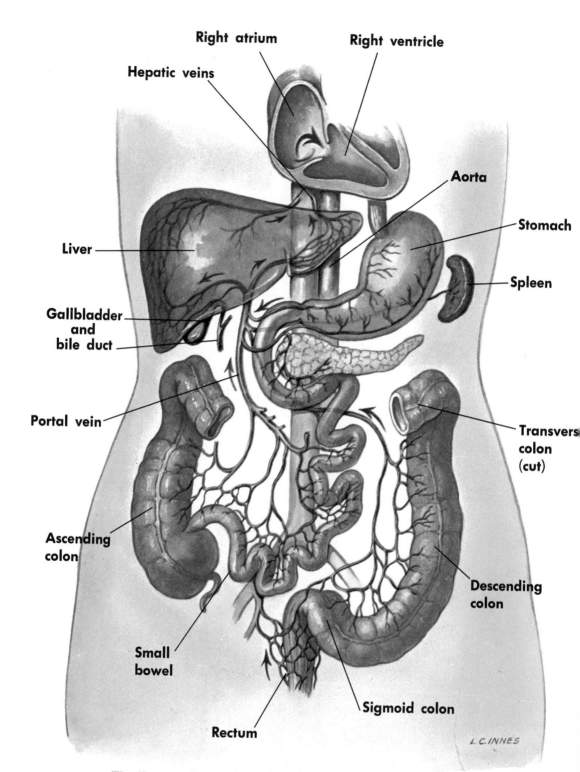

Right atrium

Right ventricle

Hepatic veins

Aorta

Liver

Stomach

Spleen

Gallbladder
and
bile duct

Portal vein

Transverse
colon
(cut)

Ascending
colon

Descending
colon

Small
bowel

Sigmoid colon

Rectum

L. C. INNES

The liver receives through the portal vein the blood that comes
from the intestines (shown in blue) laden with newly absorbed food.

343

# The Body's Covering

When the teacher asked Johnny the purpose of the skin, he responded, "The skin keeps the body from looking raw." And Johnny was right.

The skin serves as a barrier between the atmosphere that surrounds the body and the tissue fluids within. Being on the body's surface, the skin prevents the movement of fluid in either direction. It also prevents the entry into the body of irritating dusts, chemicals, and germs.

But the skin is more than a tight-fitting envelope. It helps control the body's temperature. It contains the sense organs for touch, for heat and cold, for pain, and for the feeling of pressure. The skin contains many small glands which discharge their fluid or oil onto the body's surface. Furthermore, the skin can repair itself following injury.

No single description applies to the skin of all parts of the body. Its features in one location differ from those in another. It is modified for protection against heavy friction on the palms of the hands and soles of the feet, for flexibility around the joints and parts of the body which move freely, for remarkable sensitivity around the face and other parts of the body where sense perception is important, and for the growth of hair in those areas where hair provides added protection or im-

proves a person's appearance.

In all parts of the body, however, the skin has two principal layers—a surface layer of closely packed cells (the epidermis) and a deeper layer of strong fibers arranged in a feltwork (dermis or corium).

The epidermis contains no blood vessels—just layers of closely packed cells. The deepest of these cells are very much alive and keep producing more cells just like themselves. As new cells develop, they crowd their way toward the surface, meanwhile moving farther away from their source of nourishment and undergoing chemical changes which make them horny and scalelike. When they reach the surface, they are no longer alive and eventually rub off by friction with the towel after bathing or by coming in contact with some unyielding surface. The thickness of the epidermis is greatest in those parts of the body exposed to wear and tear. A person walking barefoot develops a thick epidermis on the soles of his feet. A person whose shoe pinches develops thick areas (calluses) at the points of friction with his shoe. A violinist forms a thick epidermis on the parts of his fingers that press against the strings. The skin of the eyelids has such a thin epidermis that it is very sensitive to touch.

The deeper layer of the skin, the

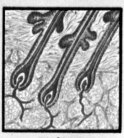
10 hairs

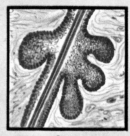
12 sebaceous
glands

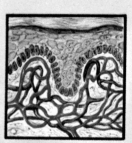
1 yard of blood vessels

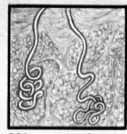
100 sweat glands

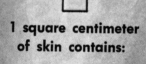
1 square centimeter
of skin contains:

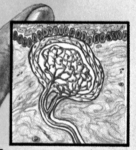
3,000,000 cells

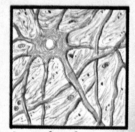
4 yards of nerves

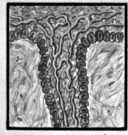
12 sensory apparatuses
for heat

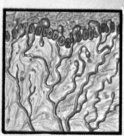
3,000 sensory cells
at the ends of
nerve fibers

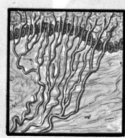
200 nerve endings
to record pain

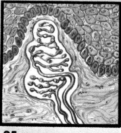
25 pressure
apparatuses for
the perception
of tactile stimuli

2 sensory apparatuses
for cold

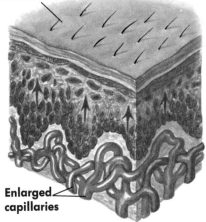

Corneum

Melanin
granules

Capillaries

Skin reddened

Enlarged
capillaries

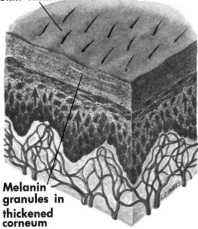

Skin tanned

Melanin
granules in
thickened
corneum

**Effects of exposure of skin to sunlight: upper, normal skin; middle, twenty-four hours after exposure (redness from blood-filled capillaries); lower, one week after exposure (tan coloration due to increase in granules of melanin).**

ultraviolet range) is produced artificially in the popular suntanning salons. It is just as damaging to the skin as the ultraviolet portion of sunlight. Persons of blond complexion, persons living in areas where the sunlight is intense (as Arizona, Texas, and Florida), and those who work continuously outdoors are the most susceptible to the skin damage caused by the ultraviolet component of sunlight.

Physicians who specialize in care of the skin recommend caution regarding exposure to the sun. They advise against patronizing the suntan salon, and they urge those who must be in the sun a great deal to protect the skin of the exposed areas by the use of a sunscreen ointment. Sunscreen ointments are available at the drugstore and do not require a prescription.

### Dry Skin

Soaps, solvents, and some disinfectants have the effect of removing the natural oil from the skin. When such are used excessively or continuously, the skin becomes dry and chapped. Exposure to dry air or to cold winds also removes the natural oil from between the surface cells of the epidermis.

Avoiding the excessive use of soap when washing the skin or bathing helps to prevent such drying. For persons living in cold climates, protective clothing (including scarves, gloves, and mittens) plus the use of humidifiers in living quarters will help to prevent dry and chapped skin.

Once the skin becomes dry because of the loss of its natural oil, the best treatment consists of soaking the involved area in warm water for five to ten minutes, following which a greasy ointment, such as petrolatum (Vaseline) or lanolin, should be rubbed into the skin. Creams and lotions for the treatment of dry skin are also available at the drugstore. Some of these consist of an emulsion designed to leave a thin film of oil on the skin.

### Hair and Nails

Each individual hair is the product of

357

# Skin Diseases

The skin is commonly affected in ways that bring discomfort and concern. It is estimated that 10 to 15 percent of patient visits to physicians are prompted by some skin ailment.

Because of its exposed position as it covers the body's surface, the skin is commonly damaged by trauma and by contact with various physical agents. It often becomes involved by infections caused by bacteria, fungi, yeasts, parasites, and viruses. It is susceptible to inflammations, to allergic reactions, and even to the development of cancer. The skin may be involved by certain systemic diseases. Some skin diseases are caused by inherited predisposi-

tions, and for some the cause has not been determined.

It is the purpose of the present chapter to systematize the present knowledge on skin diseases so that the reader can find answers to his questions on the characteristics of the common skin ailments, their causes when known, and the most successful procedures for treatment. The chapter is organized according to the following outline. Each subdivision includes detailed discussions of the individual skin diseases belonging to each respective category. To locate the discussion for a particular disease consult the index following the outline or use the General Index.

## Outline of the Chapter

| | | |
|---|---|---|
| A. AILMENTS THAT ITCH (PRURITUS) | | 363-365 |
| B. DERMATITIS | | 365-368 |
| C. BACTERIAL INFECTIONS | | 368-372 |
| D. FUNGAL INFECTIONS | | 372-374 |
| E. PARASITIC INFECTIONS | | 374-377 |
| F. VIRAL INFECTIONS | | 377-379 |
| G. DISORDERS OF HAIR FOLLICLES AND SEBACEOUS GLANDS | | 379-381 |
| H. SCALING PAPULAR DISEASES | | 381-383 |
| I. INFLAMMATORY SKIN REACTIONS | | 383-386 |
| J. PEMPHIGUS | | 386, 387 |

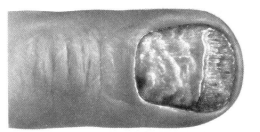

Onychomycosis. From
fungi invasion.

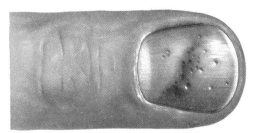

Psoriasis. Note
typical depressions.

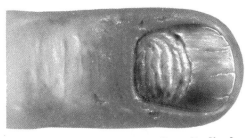

Eczema. Longitudinal
splitting distinctive.

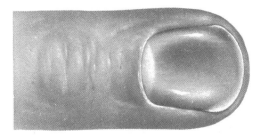

Koilonychia. Gives
"spoon nail" effect.

remove a considerable portion of the affected nail and then use medications more potent than for the usual manifestations of fungus disease. When eczema (dermatitis) affects the nails, soothing lotions usually prove helpful. The more potent forms of treatment, such as the corticosteroid medications, are used only under a physician's supervision.

Sometimes simply anointing the nails nightly with olive or castor oil will help toughen them, especially if dressings are applied to keep the oil from being rubbed off during sleep. The following cream, which should be applied every night, is better than oil in some cases:

| | |
|---|---|
| Lanolin | 1 |
| White wax | 1 |
| White petrolatum | 2 |
| Triethanolamine | 3 |
| Water q.s.ad. | 30 |

## INGROWING TOENAIL

In this condition the skin and flesh at one or both corners of the nail, usually the nail of the great toe, become tender and inflamed. The difficulty is usually caused by the wearing of shoes which force the toes into a crowded position.

### Care and Treatment

In a mild case of ingrown toenail it is usually sufficient to use a probe to clean away the cuticle debris that has accumulated along the edges of the nail plate, making sure in the meantime, that no sliver or spur at the forward corner of the nail plate is gouging into the fleshy tissue. If such a sliver or spur is present, it should be removed by scissors. Attention should also be given to selecting the kind of footwear that allows sufficient room for the toes.

For the more severe case of ingrown toenail, in which the tissues have become inflamed or infected, it is desirable to work a small wisp of cotton under the edge of the nail plate, after loosening the tissues as described above, and moisten this wisp of cotton

K. DISORDERS OF CORNIFICATION     387, 388

L. ULCERS     388-390

M. PIGMENTARY DISORDERS     390-392

N. DISORDERS OF SWEATING     392

O. SKIN REACTIONS TO LIGHT AND TEMPERATURE     392-396

P. URTICARIA (HIVES)     396, 397

Q. NAIL DISORDERS     397-399

R. BENIGN TUMORS     399-401

S. MALIGNANT CHANGES     401, 402

# Index of Skin Disorders

Acne 379
  rosacea 379
  vulgaris 379
Actinic keratosis 393, 394
Albinism 390
Alopecia 379, 380
  areata 380, 381
Ancylostomiasis 3:308, 309
Angioedema 397
Angioneurotic edema 397
Anhidrosis 392
Athlete's foot 372, 373
Atopic dermatitis 367
Bacterial infections 368-372
Baldness 379, 380
Barber's itch 373
Bedsore 389
Birthmark 399
Blackheads 1:264, 265
Body lice 376, 377
Boils 369, 370
Bromhidrosis 392
Burns 395
Callus 387, 388
Cancer 401, 402
Candidiasis 374
Carbuncles 370
Cellulitis 370, 371
Chafing 387
Chancre 473
Chancroid 475
Chilblains 395, 396
Chloasma 391
Cold injury 395, 396
Cold sore 378
Comedones 1:265
Condylomata acuminatum 378, 379
Contact dermatitis 365, 366
Corn 387, 388
Cornification disorders 387, 388
Crab lice 377
Crotch itch 374
Cyst, sebaceous 400, 401
Dandruff 367, 368
Decubitus ulcer 389
Dermatitis, atopic 367
  contact 365, 366
  exfoliative 367
  medicamentosa 383, 384

seborrheic 367, 368
  stasis 368
Dermatophytosis 372
Diabetic ulcer 389
Diaper rash 1:71
Drug rash 383, 384
Eczema 367
  involving the nails 398
Edema, angioneurotic 397
Ephelides 391
Erysipelas 371
Erythema multiforme 384, 385
  nodosum 384
Erythrasma 371
Erythroderma 367
Exfoliative dermatitis 367
Fatty tumor 401
Fever blister 378
Fishskin disease 388
Folliculitis 369
Freckles 391
Freezing Injury 396
Frostbite 396
Fungal infections 372-374
Furuncles 369, 370
Genital herpes simplex 471, 472
Genital warts 378, 379
Granuloma inguinale 475, 476
Gray hair 391
Ground itch 3:308, 309
Hair, gray 391
  loss of 379, 380
  superfluous 358, 359
  unwanted 358, 359
Hangnail 399
Head lice 376
Heat rash 1:71
Hemangioma 399
Herpes simplex 377, 378
  genital 471, 472
Herpes zoster 1:371; 3:58, 260, 261
Hirsutism 2:358
Hives 396, 397
Hookworm infection 3:308, 309
Hyperhidrosis 392
Ichthyosis 388
Impetigo 371, 372
Inflammatory diseases 383-386
Ingrowing toenail 398, 399

Intertrigo 387
Itch, "the itch" 375, 376
Itching, in the anal region 364, 365
  general 363, 364
Jock itch 374
Keloid 401
Keratosis. actinic 393, 394
  seborrheic 400
  solar 393, 394
Lesions 362, 363
Letigines, senile 391
Leukoderma 390, 391
Lice 376, 377
Lichen planus 381
Light sensitivity 394, 395
Lipoma 401
Liver spots 391
Louse infestation 376, 377
Lupus erythematosus 385, 386
Lymphogranuloma venereum 476
Medicamentosa dermatitis 383, 384
Melanoma 402
Melasma 391
Miliaria 394
Mole 399, 400
Moniliasis 374
Nail disorders 397-399
Parasitic infections 374-377
Paronychia 399
Pediculosis 376, 377
  capitis 376
  corporis 376, 377
  pubis 377
Pemphigus 386, 387
Perspiratory disorders 392
Photosensitivity 394, 395
Pigmentary disorders 390-392
Pityriasis rosea 381
Plantar wart 378
Poison ivy 366, 367
Poison oak 366, 367
Prickly heat 394
Pruritus ani 364, 365
Pruritus, general 363, 364
Psoriasis, general 382, 383
  involving the nails 398
Rash, definition and significance 362
  diaper 1:71
  heat 1:71

every few hours with a saturated solution of Epsom salts.

The use of an alternating hot and cold footbath each morning and evening, as described in chapter 25, volume 3, is helpful in relieving pain and inflammation. For cases in which the pain and infection become extreme, it may be necessary to have the physician remove a slender, lengthwise strip of the nail plate in the involved area.

## PARONYCHIA

In paronychia the tissues which surround the fingernails, or occasionally, the toenails, become infected. The involved tissues are swollen and extremely tender and may exude pus. In the most persistent cases, the nail plate becomes thickened and discolored with transverse ridges. Often, several fingers are involved at the same time.

Paronychia usually develops in persons whose hands are immersed in water a great deal. In such, a slight injury to the finger allows bacteria or fungi to invade the tissues surrounding the nail. The susceptibility is greater in persons with diabetes or those whose nutrition is deficient.

### Care and Treatment

Avoid as much as possible immersing the hands in water. After washing the hands, dry the fingers gently and thoroughly. When it becomes necessary to immerse the hands (as when washing dishes), wear cotton gloves next to the skin and cover these with rubber gloves. Before retiring at night, apply a medicated cream to the fingers, working it carefully into the tissues surrounding the fingernails. Suitable preparations for this condition include these: (1) Mycolog cream and (2) Castellani paint (carbolfuchsin solution). For a persisting troublesome infection, the physician may prescribe an antibiotic medication.

## HANGNAIL

Sometimes the cuticle which surrounds the nail at its base splits and creates a fissure which tears into the living tissue. The area becomes painful and may even be infected.

### Care and Treatment

Gently trimming away the loosened tissue will usually allow the fissure to heal. For prevention, it is advisable to use a mild cream, massaging it into the nail margins so as to keep these tissues pliable.

# R. Benign Tumors

## BIRTHMARK (HEMANGIOMA, VASCULAR NEVUS)

Inasmuch as birthmarks appear in early life, this blemish of the skin is considered in chapter 17, volume 1.

## MOLES (NEVI)

Practically everyone has at least a few moles located here and there in the skin. A mole develops even before birth as a cluster of melanocytes—the cells capable of producing the pigment melanin. Many moles do not become apparent until adulthood, even though their basic cells were present from before birth. In some moles, practically no melanin is produced, and therefore the mole remains the color of the surrounding skin. In others, the pigment melanin accounts for varying degrees

Some moles may become cancerous.

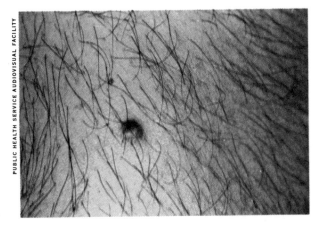

PUBLIC HEALTH SERVICE AUDIOVISUAL FACILITY

of darkness, even up to a purple-black color.

The possibility that a mole may, in an occasional case, transform into a malignant tumor is considered under the heading of Melanoma, in the next section of this chapter, page 402.

### Care and Treatment

Except for the occasional possibility of a developing melanoma, as suggested in the previous paragraph, moles are harmless and require no treatment. Some persons desire that a mole appearing in a conspicuous place be removed. This can be done in a doctor's office by a simple procedure. Moles subject to irritation from clothing, such as at the belt line or under a bra strap should preferably be removed by the doctor even though, as yet, they may not show any tendency to be troublesome.

### SEBORRHEIC KERATOSIS

Seborrheic keratosis is a condition in which many, small, slightly-raised lesions develop on the skin of a middle-aged or elderly person. The lesions are simple tumors, but they are not dangerous. They are not malignant and they have no tendency to become so. They are the most common type of skin tumor occurring in elderly persons.

The lesions of seborrheic keratosis are usually numerous. They occur on the face, including the forehead, on the neck, on the chest, and on the back. They vary in size, even in the same person, from a few millimeters in diameter to as much as several centimeters across. Most commonly they are only slightly darker than the surrounding skin, but some may be dark brown, even black. They are round (or oval) and are sharply demarcated from the surrounding skin. They are covered with a loosely attached, greasy crust. When the crust is removed, the base appears raw and pulpy and bleeds slightly. The surface of the lesion is smooth and shiny and may be crisscrossed by clefts. The lesion is soft and can be rolled between the fingers.

The lesions of seborrheic keratosis produce no symptoms except itching which, in some cases, is intense.

### Care and Treatment

It is important for the person with skin lesions such as described above to see his doctor for a positive diagnosis. The lesions of a more serious skin condition may be mistaken for those of seborrheic keratosis. Once the diagnosis of seborrheic keratosis is confirmed, the only reason for the lesions to be removed is to relieve the itching, if present, or for cosmetic reasons. The lesions can be removed by a simple surgical procedure which leaves little or no scar.

### SEBACEOUS CYST (WEN)

A sebaceous cyst is a harmless growth which results from the plugging of the outlet of a sebaceous gland—the oil gland associated with a hair follicle. Even with its outlet plugged, the gland continues to secrete the kind of oily material which it normally produces. Thus there develops a sac filled with an

**Sebaceous cyst, called a wen, commonly appears on the neck or face.**

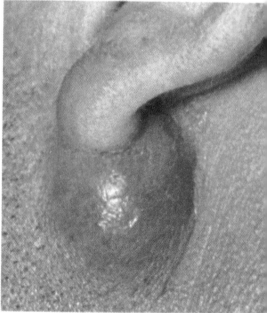

PUBLIC HEALTH SERVICE AUDIOVISUAL FACIL

breast. A bloody discharge sometimes accompanies benign conditions, but it also occurs in certain cases of cancer of the breast.

2. *Pain in the Breast.* Many women experience mild discomfort in the breasts prior to each menstrual period. Significant pain in the breast is noticed, of course, when an infection develops (mastitis) and in some cases of mammary dysplasia. Early cancer of the breast is usually not accompanied by pain. Perhaps this is unfortunate, for the absence of pain may be falsely reassuring to the woman with an early cancer of the breast.

3. *Changes in Appearance.* In many healthy women one breast is slightly higher than the other and this should cause no concern. But when a change occurs in the shape or appearance of a breast it should be examined by a physician to determine whether disease is developing. Retraction or deviation of one nipple as compared with the other should raise a woman's suspicion. Also, the dimpling of skin over any part of the breast is probably caused by the development of an abnormal condition within the breast.

4. *Detection of a lump.* A woman should make a self-examination of her breasts at least every month. The method of performing this is explained in chapter 11, volume 3, where there is a detailed discussion of cancer of the breast. Many times a lump in the breast is caused by a benign form of disease. However, a lump in the breast is often the first evidence of cancer. Therefore, the finding of a lump in the breast should be taken very seriously, and professional advice should be obtained at once.

## ACUTE MASTITIS (INFLAMMATION OF THE BREAST)

Acute mastitis is an infection usually caused by invasion of the staphylococcus germ through a fissure in the delicate skin that covers the nipple. The in-fection typically occurs a few days or a few weeks after childbirth in a case where the mother is nursing her infant. The infection tends to find its way into some particular area of the breast. The skin over this area becomes red, tender, and firm to the touch.

In the early stage of this infection, the progress of the infection can be halted by the appropriate use of antibiotic medication. When the infection is allowed to progress, the patient develops fever, and a strong possibility exists that an abscess will develop within the breast. Once an abscess forms, a surgical incision must be made so that the abscess can be drained.

When the infection is controlled reasonably early by antibiotic medication, it is acceptable for the infant to continue drawing milk from this breast.

## MAMMARY DYSPLASIA (CHRONIC CYSTIC MASTITIS)

This is a condition in which cystic (hollow, fluid-filled) nodules develop within the breast. The condition develops in about 20 percent of women in the 30-to-50 age bracket. It usually involves both breasts, and the cystic nodules of varying sizes are easily felt by the examining fingers.

There may be no symptoms other than the discovery of the nodules, but in many cases pain or tenderness call attention to the presence of these nodules. There may be a slight discharge from the nipple. In some cases, the cysts tend to enlarge just before the time of menstruation. The exact cause of mammary dysplasia is not known, but the fact that the cysts tend to disappear at the time of the menopause without later recurrence, suggests that their development is caused by an imbalance of the endocrine system.

Mammary dysplasia, of itself, is harmless except for the inconvenience and discomfort. But the seriousness of this condition is that it may be easily confused with beginning cancer of the breast. It is tragic, of course, when a beginning cancer is mistakenly considered to be mammary dysplasia and

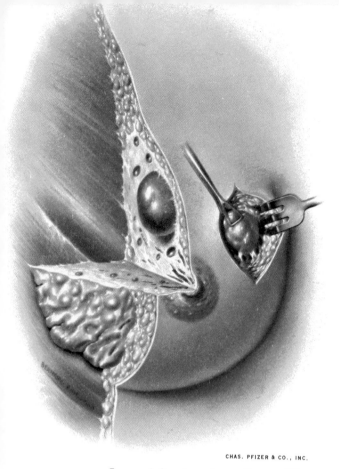

Lower left, chronic cystic mastitis; center, cystic disease with single large cyst; right, benign tumor.

valuable time is lost for treating the cancer. The findings on examination of the breast in mammary dysplasia resemble those in cancer so closely that it is imperative when lumps develop within the breast to make sure which condition is present. This certainty is accomplished by the minor surgical procedure of removing one or more of the lumps for microscopic examination.

### Care and Treatment

Once it is made certain that the condition in the breast is that of mammary dysplasia, the larger lumps can be reduced by the physician inserting a small needle and withdrawing the fluid which the cysts contain. Also, appropriate endocrine preparations may reduce the cyst formation. Oral

contraceptives, containing hormones as they do, may be of help. Even so, the patient with mammary dysplasia should be examined at frequent intervals (every six months) as a means of detecting any development of cancer. The woman with mammary dysplasia carries twice the prospect of developing cancer of the breast as does the woman without mammary dysplasia. The pain and the tenderness associated with the presence of cysts in this disease can be partially relieved by the wearing of a brassiere which gives good support and protects, somewhat from mechanical injury.

### FIBROADENOMA

A fibroadenoma is a true tumor of the breast, a disease slightly less common than cancer of the breast. It tends to occur in relatively young women—in the 15- to 35-year age group. It is not classed as malignant, because it does not tend to spread. It typically occurs as a single, round, rubbery, painless mass which may be up to two inches (5 cm.) in diameter. A fibroadenoma may increase in size during a pregnancy.

### Care and Treatment

The treatment for a fibroadenoma is surgical removal of the tumor. This is accomplished rather simply because this type of tumor is enclosed within a capsule of fibrous tissue.

### CANCER OF THE BREAST

Cancer of the breast is considered in chapter 11, volume 3. It is a serious disease because of the tendency to spread to other parts of the body. Cancer of the breast is highly malignant. It occurs quite commonly, involving, on the average, one out of every thirteen Caucasian women. Many studies have been made to determine what factors predominate in making a woman susceptible to this disease. In summary, cancer of the breast occurs most commonly under the following conditions.

1. Caucasian race.
2. Age above 50.

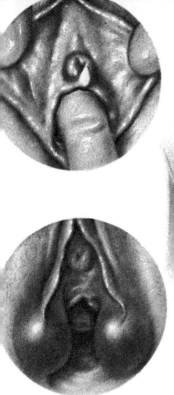

 appears throughout the top left illustrations.

A. Sectional view of female sex organs, showing possible complications of nonspecific urethritis: urethritis, vaginitis, endometritis (inflammation within the uterus), and salpingitis. B. Glands in the wall of urethra become involved in inflammation of urethritis. C. Glands in wall of vulva frequently become inflamed as a complication of urethritis.

above, some physicians prescribe a single, large dose (2 grams) of metronidazole (Flagyl).

## VAGINAL FISTULAS

A fistula is an abnormal opening between two structures. A vaginal fistula may consist of an opening between the vagina and the bladder, between the vagina and the urethra, or between the vagina and the rectum. Such fistulas develop as the result of accidents, infections, abscesses, radiation burns, or tissue damage such as sometimes occurs at childbirth. When the fistula extends between the vagina and the urinary organs, urine will dribble from the vagina. When the fistula is between the vagina and the rectum, fecal material may seep into the vagina from the rectum.

### Care and Treatment

The treatment of vaginal fistula consists of a plastic surgical procedure in which the damaged tissues are repaired so that the abnormal connection is obliterated.

## F. Vulvar Diseases

The vulva is the region of the external sex organs of the female. It includes the labia major and minor, the area and space between the labia (the vestibule), and the skin immediately surrounding the labia. In the present section we consider the common disorders that may affect the region of the vulva.

### VULVAR PRURITUS

Pruritus (itching) of the delicate skin in the region of the vulva is one of the most common symptoms relating to the female sex organs. Notice that this is a symptom, not a disease. There are many possible causes, and in order to relieve the symptom the cause must be determined and the treatment arranged accordingly. We now list the several common causes of vulvar pruritus, along with care and remedies:

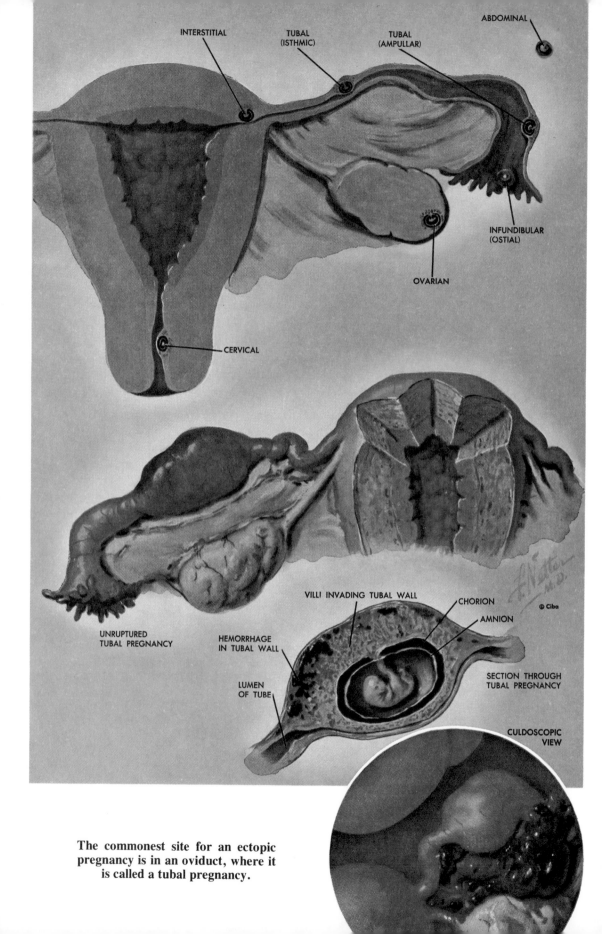

INTERSTITIAL

TUBAL (ISTHMIC)

TUBAL (AMPULLAR)

ABDOMINAL

INFUNDIBULAR (OSTIAL)

OVARIAN

CERVICAL

UNRUPTURED TUBAL PREGNANCY

VILLI INVADING TUBAL WALL

CHORION

AMNION

HEMORRHAGE IN TUBAL WALL

SECTION THROUGH TUBAL PREGNANCY

LUMEN OF TUBE

CULDOSCOPIC VIEW

The commonest site for an ectopic pregnancy is in an oviduct, where it is called a tubal pregnancy.

an's birth canal is unavoidable at the time of childbirth. The tissues are more or less bruised, stretched, and torn. But with good obstetrical care the amount of laceration is usually so slight that it can be successfully repaired, if necessary, by a few stitches taken immediately after the delivery of the child. But in spite of the best of care, bad lacerations, involving even the tissues of the perineum (the pelvic floor), sometimes occur. The severity of the damage may not be apparent until a thorough examination is made a few weeks after delivery.

When repair of the tissues of the birth canal or the perineum is neglected, there develops a loss of support of the pelvic organs, a problem that gives rise to such symptoms as a feeling of heaviness in the pelvis, pain in the vicinity of the ovaries, headache, general lassitude, physical debility, nervousness, and constipation. The uterus is usually in an abnormal position, pulling on some of the organs surrounding it and pressing on others. In extreme cases, the uterus may have sagged down to such an extent that the cervix protrudes from the vagina. Straining at stool may cause the rectum to pouch into the vagina, producing what is called rectocele. The lack of proper support may allow the bladder to pouch in front of the vagina, producing what is called cystocele. This interferes with the proper emptying of the bladder and cystitis may result.

### Care and Treatment

**In mild cases of relaxation of the pelvic supports, exercises such as are described in the item that follows will serve to strengthen the muscles in the perineum and relieve whatever symptoms may occur in these mild cases. In the more extensive cases in which rectocele and/or cystocele have developed, it is advisable to consult a physician, preferably a gynecologist, who will make a careful examination and recommend a procedure of surgical repair. Such surgery does not require that the abdomen be opened, but it does involve the use of a general anesthetic and plastic surgical procedure to return the organs and muscles of the pelvic region to their normal position.**

### VAGINAL (PUBOCOCCYGEAL) EXERCISES

Many physicians are now recommending a simple exercise procedure to their women patients to strengthen the muscles and tone up the tissues of the perineum (in the region of the vagina). These exercises are especially beneficial (1) after childbirth, (2) in a case of urinary incontinence (dribbling of urine), (3) before surgery for the repair of old perineal lacerations, and (4) in a case in which sex relations are hindered because of the chronic relaxation of the perineal tissues.

The exercise is performed twice each day (morning and evening). It consists of voluntary tensing of the muscles at the outlet of the vagina as in the effort to prevent the flow of urine. The muscle tension is maintained for about six seconds, followed by relaxation for six seconds. The 12-second sequence is repeated 12 to 24 times at each session.

# Sexually Transmitted Diseases

The tissues of the sex organs are delicate. The exposed areas are invested by thin skin and the concealed portions are bounded by fragile, moist membranes. The delicacy of these tissues makes it easy for germs to invade and propagate there in a warm, moist environment. There are several types of disease-producing germs that not only thrive in these tissues but may spread to other tissues, even throughout the body in some cases, causing serious destruction of tissues as they spread. The consequences are often tragic, causing suffering, pathetic damage to unborn children, inability to become parents, and even premature death.

The diseases caused by the germs of which we speak here are contagious diseases, easily transmitted when one person's sex organs come in contact with the corresponding areas of another person's body. Thus we speak of these diseases as sexually transmitted diseases.

Once one of these diseases becomes established in a person's body, it tends to persist, if untreated, for the duration of life. Some persons so afflicted have obvious symptoms and some do not. In some of these diseases the symptoms are present only at certain periods. Most victims of these diseases become infected with them without their knowledge.

Effective remedies are now available for most of the sexually transmitted diseases (not so for genital herpes simplex); but the number of cases has increased alarmingly, even so, and many cases still go untreated. Because these diseases are often acquired under clandestine circumstances, many sufferers are reluctant to seek treatment.

Analysts propose various reasons for the tremendous increase in recent years of the sexually transmitted diseases: Many returning war veterans brought these diseases with them. Popular methods of contraception, reducing the fear of unwanted pregnancy, have encouraged sexual promiscuity. Deteriorating moral standards have tempted many to be permissive regarding premarital and extramarital sexual intercourse. Many present-day teenagers allow themselves to be influenced by the loose morality portrayed on screen and tube. Increased use of drugs and liquor weakens inhibitions to engage in intimate conduct.

The following descriptions of the common sexually transmitted diseases are arranged in groups according to the obvious signs or evidences of the particular diseases: (A) those causing an

have entered, they not only multiply in the local tissues at the site of entrance, but they travel through the lymphatic vessels and blood channels throughout the body. But this early dissemination of the germs causes no symptoms. The first discernible evidence that an infection has occurred is the appearance of a single papule at the site of entrance, which then ulcerates to form the so-called chancre or primary lesion.

The chancre is a round ulcer with raised edges and a firm texture. It varies in size, being as small as one fourth inch (6 mm.) in diameter in some cases or as large as three fourths inch (19 mm.) in diameter in others. It is painless. Usually there is just one. In women the chancre typically occurs in the vagina or on the cervix of the uterus. In men it occurs usually on the skin of the penis. It may occur in the mouth in either sex. A chancre tends to heal spontaneously in one to six weeks, but this does not mean that the disease has abated. It only means that the disease is progressing from its primary stage (the stage of the chancre) to its secondary stage. The disease is extremely contagious during this primary stage, for the ulcerated area of the chancre contains many germs.

If the person infected with syphilis has not been adequately treated during the primary stage, the evidences of the secondary stage begin about six weeks after the chancre heals. These consist of multiple lesions on the skin and membranes, plus enlargement of the lymph nodes and one or more of various problems in the internal organs and nervous system.

The so-called mucocutaneous lesions (in membranes and skin) of the secondary stage constitute a generalized rash which lasts for two to six weeks. Pink macules appear in the skin and membranes, often even of the palms and soles. The scalp is often affected with a resulting spotty loss of hair—a "moth-eaten alopecia." Round, slightly raised, painless gray plaques appear on the lips, in the mouth, and on the delicate skin of the vulva or of the glans of

the penis. Even though these skin lesions heal within a few weeks, they tend to recur one or more times in about one fourth of cases. These lesions contain the germs of syphilis, and thus the condition continues to be contagious. The various organs that may be affected during this secondary stage include the spleen, the liver, the meninges, and the eye.

Following the secondary stage, syphilis becomes quiescent for a variable time in the so-called latent stage. Early in this latent stage there may be a transient return of the mucocutaneous lesions which characterize the secondary stage. The disease may continue to be contagious during the first four years or so of this latent stage. For the most part the person is symptom-free during this time, even though the germs of syphilis are still present in his tissues.

In the untreated case this latent period may be as short as two years or it may last for the remainder of life. In the usual case it is followed in about twenty years by the late stage (tertiary stage) in which serious, destructive lesions develop in the nervous system and/or in the cardiovascular system.

In about one fourth of untreated cases the germs of syphilis invade the nervous system during the secondary stage of the disease (from three to eighteen months after the infection is acquired). The germs lie dormant here throughout the latent phase only to cause such tragic complications as general paresis and tabes dorsalis during the late stage of the disease. For a description of these complications, see the section on "Syphilis of the Nervous System," in chapter 4, volume 3.

Complications of late syphilis affecting the cardiovascular system cause a destructive process in the tissues of the first portion of the aorta, resulting in aortitis, thoracic aortic aneurysm, and aortic insufficiency of the heart.

Another dreadful manifestation of untreated syphilis is its involvement of the unborn child. The fetus is not susceptible to the syphilis which may be

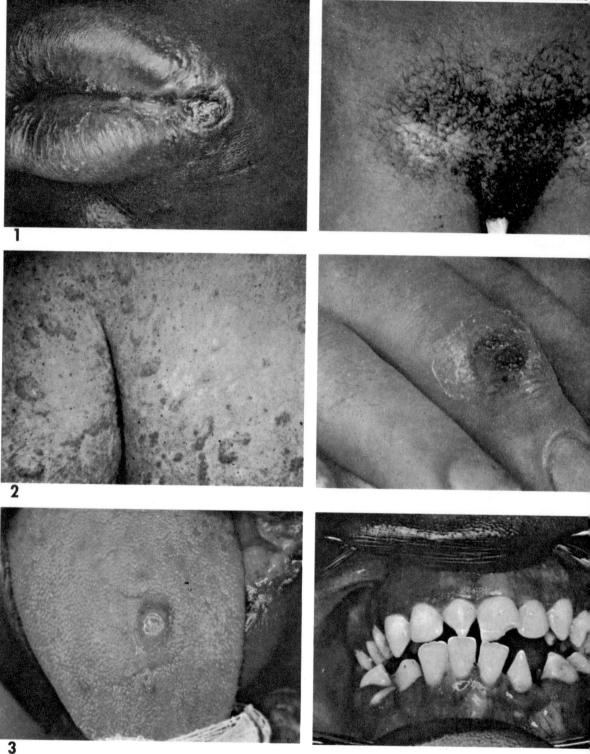

Manifestations of syphilis as they appear on various parts of the body: (1) chancre on the lip; (2) blotches on the skin; (3) chancre on the tongue; (4) swollen lymph nodes of the groin; (5) chancre on finger; and (6) notched, peg-shaped teeth (the latter a condition typical of syphilis acquired prior to birth).

# PROMINENT ACHIEVEMENTS IN MEDICINE

*(a pictorial supplement)*

Medical practice keeps moving from the past and present to the future tense. In a world where knowledge doubles at least every seven years, it is not surprising that medicine too is in the midst of an information explosion.

Physicians and medical educators who gaze into the crystal ball see amazing new developments in the offing: mankind free from infectious disease, enjoyment of physical and mental life up to age ninety or a hundred, replacement of defective parts of the body with artificial devices, diagnosis by computer (even "penny-in-the-slot" medical checkups), surgery by laser beams, improvement of memory by drugs, and on and on.

But progress in medicine, whether past, present, or future, is and always will be associated with individual men and women—gifted people who rise to prominence and contribute of their talents to the betterment of their fellows. Illustrious and long is the roster of names of people who have thus contributed, and the list continues to grow.

Readers of current literature have admired the biographical profiles of great people in medicine as presented by Parke, Davis & Company in their *History of Medicine in Pictures*. Reproductions of paintings in full color, and historical articles covering the history of medicine from antiquity to the present day, appeared in the company's *Therapeutic notes*, and in other magazines, beginning with 1957.

Great names responsible for great breakthroughs include Hippocrates, Galen, Vesalius, Edward Jenner, William Harvey, Philippe Pinel, Louis Pasteur, John Hunter, Benjamin Rush, and many others. Here we present paintings of seven of these persons, with a condensation of the write-up about each one. Parke, Davis & Company undertook this project as a service in behalf of the profession of medicine, and also as a means of promoting understanding and appreciation for what medicine throughout the centuries has meant to better health and welfare.

The authors and publishers of *You and Your Health* acknowledge their indebtedness to Artist Robert A. Thom for the paintings, to George A. Bender and his associates for the text, and of course to Parke, Davis & Company for permission to reproduce this material.

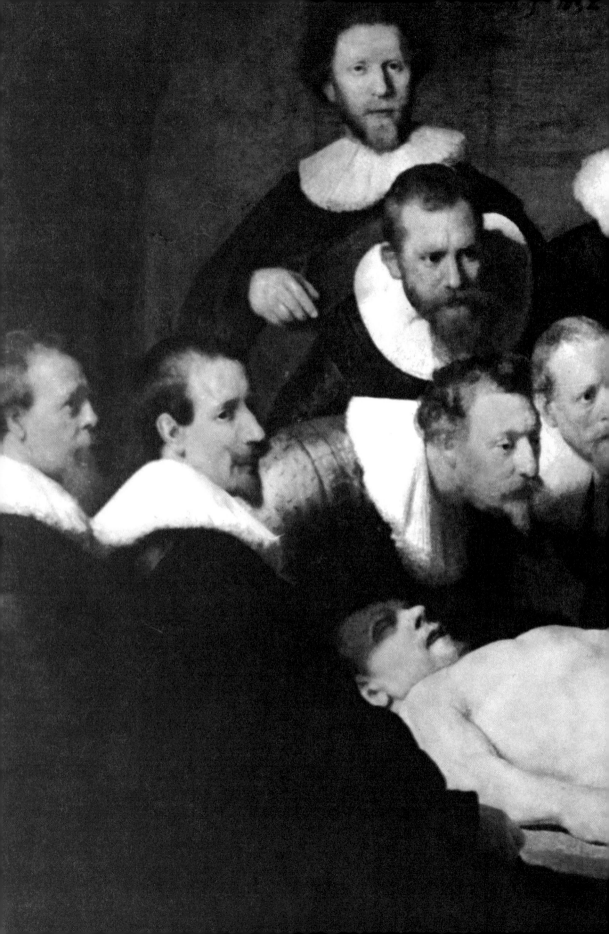

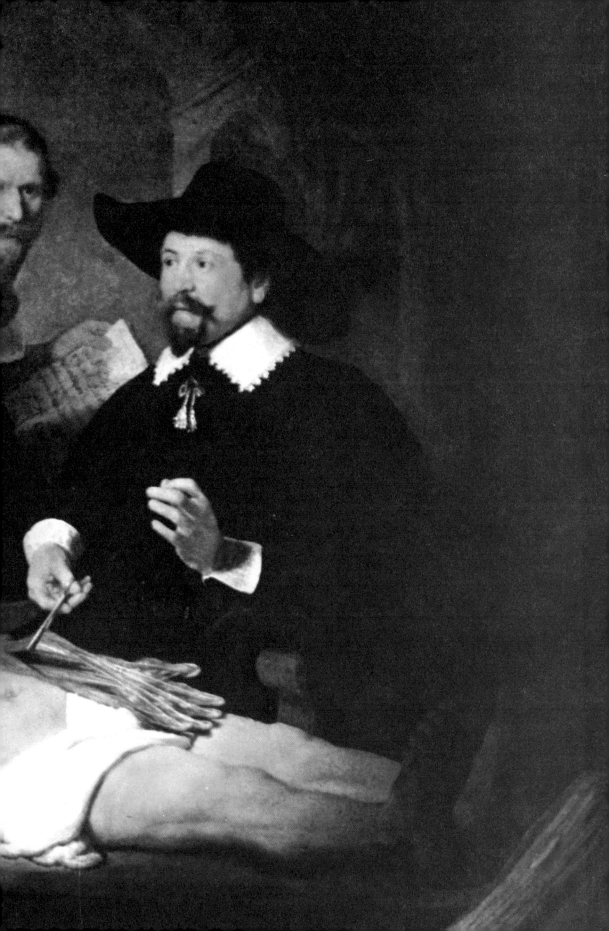

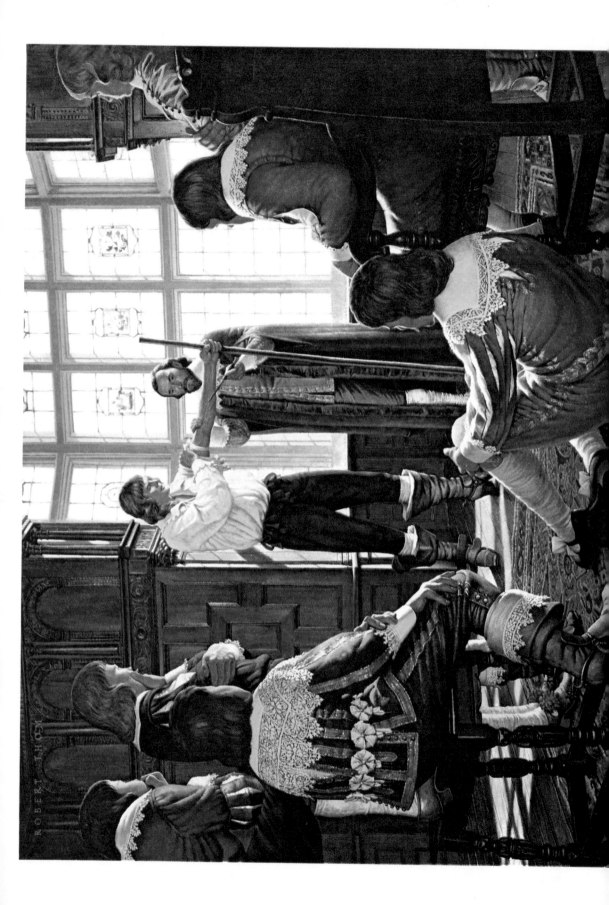

# HARVEY AND THE CIRCULATION OF THE BLOOD

William Harvey (1578-1657) demonstrated proof of his revolutionary theory of the circulation of the blood during anatomical lectures before London's College of Physicians. His *De Motu Cordis* upset Galenic tradition and introduced new concepts of anatomy.

What has been called the greatest discovery ever made in physiology—the circulation of the blood—was quietly announced early in the seventeenth century as a part of a series of lectures in anatomy. The man who brought about this discovery was William Harvey, a short, slight, dark-complexioned Englishman, with flashing, spirited eyes and a wealth of nervous energy.

William Harvey was born at Folkestone, England, April 1, 1578, the eldest son of a large well-to-do family. He was given every educational advantage and was graduated with a bachelor of arts degree from Caius College at Cambridge University in 1597. Shortly thereafter Harvey enrolled in the University of Padua's famed medical school and studied under Fabricius of Aquapendente. In later years Harvey was to acknowledge his debt to the great teacher, crediting Fabricius's work on the valves in veins for having stimulated him to investigate the mystery of blood circulation.

Harvey received the degree of doctor of medicine from the University of Padua in 1602 and returned to England the same year. Quickly rising to prominence, he was appointed physician to St. Bartholomew's Hospital in 1609 and held this important position until 1643. He also was

early elected a Fellow by the College of Physicians, and continued close association with this distinguished group throughout his life.

Harvey began his lectures on anatomy in April, 1616, in the College of Physicians' new headquarters at Amen Corner, at the end of Paternoster Row. Of great significance among his first lecture notes is the first clue to Harvey's convictions concerning blood circulation and the heart.

It was not until twelve years later, in 1628, that Harvey saw fit to publish his great work—a book which revolutionized the thinking of medical men in anatomy and therapeutics. The title: *Exercitatio Anatomica de Motu Cordis et Sanguinis in Animalibus*—"An Anatomical Treatise on the Movement of the Heart and Blood in Animals."

In essence, Harvey's observations were: The heart is a muscular organ that contracts and relaxes; at each contraction of the auricles, blood is forced into corresponding ventricles, and thence into the great arteries as the ventricles contract; once in the arteries, blood cannot return directly to the heart because of the heart valves.

Harvey's experiments were at once simple and illuminating. One was made by having an assistant grasp a staff firmly in his hand. Harvey, then, by depressing visible veins with one or two fingers, could demonstrate the single direction of flow of venous blood.

Death came to William Harvey on June 3, 1657, in his eightieth year. Thus was closed one of the most fruitful careers in medicine of the seventeenth century, contributions of which were to benefit all mankind thereafter.

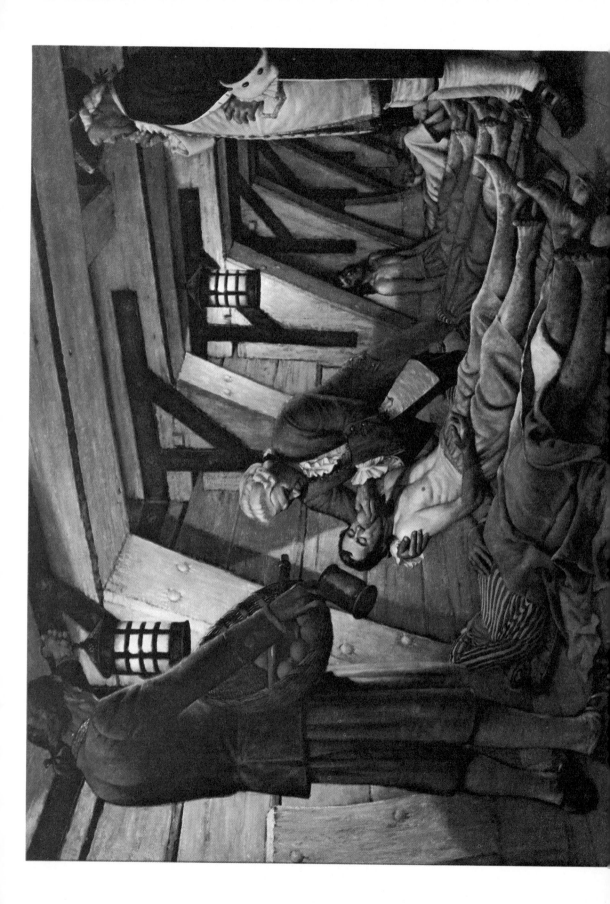

# JAMES LIND—CONQUEROR OF SCURVY

Surgeon in Britain's Royal Navy, James Lind in 1747 conducted clinical experiments proving citrus fruits would cure scurvy, dreaded killer of seamen. His recommendations and writings helped reform naval health practices.

World history and destinies of nations have been shaped on more than one occasion by alert physicians' capabilities to observe, to test, to provide solutions for health problems, and, most important of all, to convince governmental authorities that decisive remedial actions must be taken. Such a man was James Lind, naval surgeon, who pointed the way to overcome scurvy, scourge of old-time sailing ships.

Scurvy was known to and described by the ancients; but it did not assume calamitous proportions until sailing vessels replaced oared galleys, thereby making possible long journeys on the high seas. Prior to 1450, ships seldom ventured far from land, so frequent provisioning was not a problem.

It is said that, during the three centuries from 1500 to 1800, scurvy caused more deaths among sailors than other diseases, naval engagements, marine disasters, shipwrecks, and accidents combined. During this 300-year period it is estimated that not less than a million lives were taken by this dreaded form of avitaminosis, even though naval surgeons had published reports of observations relative both to means of remedy and to prevention!

James Lind, born in Edinburgh, Scotland, October 4, 1716, and educated in this famous medical center, early chose the practice of medicine as his lifework.

As did many young Scottish medical students of the period, Lind entered service in the Royal Navy as a surgeon's mate in 1739. During his ten years of service, Lind saw many men ill with scurvy. Ordinary seamen's diet was almost vitamin-free, so that after a few weeks at sea, beset by fatigue, by wetness, by cold, by loss of sleep, and by homesickness, sailors showed symptoms and signs of scurvy and of other diseases with appalling frequency.

Value of the juice of citrus fruits, of sauerkraut, of fresh vegetables, and of greens in treatment of scurvy had been recognized, and reports on success therewith published, more than a century before Lind's time; but a confusion of useless measures and recommended drugs also had developed, with the result that true remedies failed to impress most medical men. It remained for Lind, on May 20, 1747, to inaugurate a simple, straightforward series of tests, in the best clinical tradition, in order to determine relative effectiveness of half a dozen of the more popular measures. His experiments proved that citrus fruits or their juices would cure scurvy.

Dr. Lind did not live to see the Admiralty enforce the use of lemon juice as a prophylactic against scurvy (this came at the insistence of Lind's pupils, Blane and Trotter, in 1795); but he did see other recommendations put into effect to improve conditions for naval recruits.

On July 18, 1794, death came to Dr. Lind, but his influence on medical practice lives on. His work, including his three published books, had much to do with reforming naval practices, saving lives, and shaping nations' destinies.

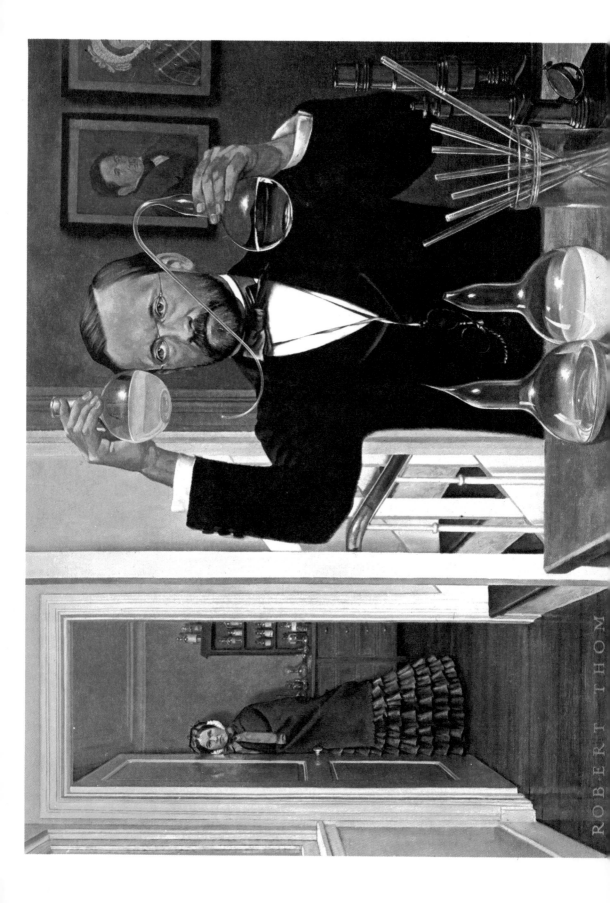

# PASTEUR: THE CHEMIST WHO TRANSFORMED MEDICINE

Practice of medicine was radically changed by experiments of France's chemist and biologist, Louis Pasteur (1822-1895). In makeshift laboratories in Paris he proved germs cause disease; that sterilization kills them; that vaccination may protect against infection.

By the middle of the nineteenth century, medical men knew but little more than had their Greek forebears about actual causes of the great scourges of the race—the plagues, the fevers, and the pestilences. At the close of the century, at the end of Pasteur's career, the germ theory had been proved and no longer was seriously contested; the patterns of many infective diseases were understood; methods had been devised for preventing or for combating some of the most serious infections; conditions under which surgical procedures were carried out had been revolutionized; and the sciences of bacteriology and of preventive medicine had been launched.

Louis Pasteur, born December 27, 1822, grew up in France, his native country, and attended the Royal College of Besançon, graduating with a baccalaureate in science in 1842, but ironically with a grade of "mediocre" in chemistry.

In September, 1848, Pasteur was appointed professor of physics at the lyceum (high school) in Dijon, but in December was promoted to be assistant professor of chemistry on the Faculty of Sciences at Strasbourg. There he married Marie Laurent, who proved to be just the kind of wife the scientist needed. She was tolerant of his devotion to research, assisted him with his notes and his records, and looked after his physical well-being during an active and hectic career.

Studies begun in 1860 in both alcoholic and lactic fermentation led Pasteur to his greatest and most revolutionary contributions to science—study and refutation of the theory of spontaneous generation, undisputable proof of the existence of germs, of their modes of reproduction, and of their specificity in causing disease. From these studies arose Pasteur's suggestion that vintners might protect their product, without injury, by heating bottled wine for several minutes at 55° C. (131° F.). Thus was the process, now called pasteurization, introduced.

Another significant achievement in the fruitful life of this great scientist was development of a prophylactic treatment against rabies—an achievement that paved the way for development of other vaccines and antitoxins. Physicians and scientists from all over the world flocked to Pasteur's laboratories to learn firsthand Pasteur's techniques and doctrines, which were rapidly revolutionizing the practice of medicine.

Pasteur's seventieth birthday was occasion for an ovation at the Sorbonne, attended by scientists and political figures from many countries. Lister paid the tribute: "Pasteur has lifted the veil that for centuries has hidden the infectious diseases."

During the next three years Pasteur's health steadily declined. After he suffered a series of cerebrovascular accidents, death came September 28, 1895.

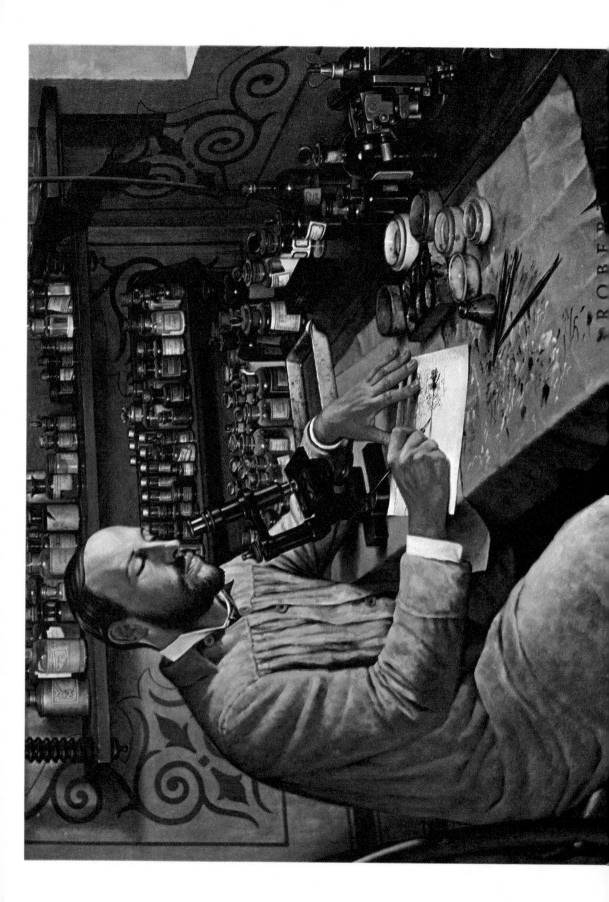

# RAMON y CAJAL: CHARTING THE NERVOUS SYSTEM

Boyhood teachers were positive that no good would come of the backward, headstrong, artistically inclined country surgeon's son Santiago Ramón y Cajal (1852-1934). However, he became Spain's leading medical scientist, world-renowned as a neuroanatomist. In 1906 he was awarded the Nobel prize in medicine.

The stern fathers at the Latin school in Jaca were agreed: Santiago Ramón y Cajal probably wouldn't amount to much. According to their report, he was a poor student; he didn't use his memory; his flair for art was used more often as an outlet for his resentments than for studious purposes; he seemed stubborn and inflexible. No amount of flogging or denial of suppers would change his ways. So, bruised and half-starved, the boy was returned to his father, a country surgeon who eked out a precarious living in the Spanish Pyrenees village of Ayerbe. The busy doctor was both furious and frustrated. He had hoped his boy would become a physician too; but perhaps, as teachers predicted, he was destined only to be a tradesman.

From such boyhood experiences came the young man who was destined to become Spain's leading scientist, histologist, neuroanatomist, and a personage revered equally by scientists, politicians, educators, and peasants.

In 1869, when Santiago was seventeen, the elder Ramón received appointment as professor of anatomy on the Faculty of Medicine at Zaragoza. He was at once filled with zeal to train his son as a skilled dissector.

In June, 1877, Santiago went to Madrid to take examinations for his doctorate in medicine. While at the university he had an experience that was to change his life: One of the professors showed him a microscope and some microscopic preparations. Intrigued, Ramón y Cajal spent his savings for a microscope, a microtome, and a few supplies.

Back at Zaragoza, Ramón y Cajal, having been appointed as instructor in anatomy and director of the Anatomical Museum, readily developed an interest in histology—the study of tissues. Later, in 1887, he was called to accept the professorship of histology at the University of Barcelona.

In Barcelona Ramón y Cajal, then thirty-five years of age, seriously began the work that was to give him distinction and to strengthen his position as a medical researcher. He began a systematic study of the entire nervous system, staining cells and tissues with a clarity which never had been achieved before. To his scientific techniques he added his talent of drawing.

Soon he became recognized internationally and gained further acceptance and appreciation at home. In 1892 he was called to assume the chair of Normal Histology and Pathological Anatomy at the University of Madrid. His findings received wide publication and acclaim.

Among Ramón y Cajal's greater contributions to medical knowledge and to the fields of neurology and psychiatry, wrote historian F. H. Garrison, were the elucidation "of the developmental and structural basis of the dynamics of the neuron; of transmission of impulse; of localization of function; and of degeneration and regeneration in the nervous system."

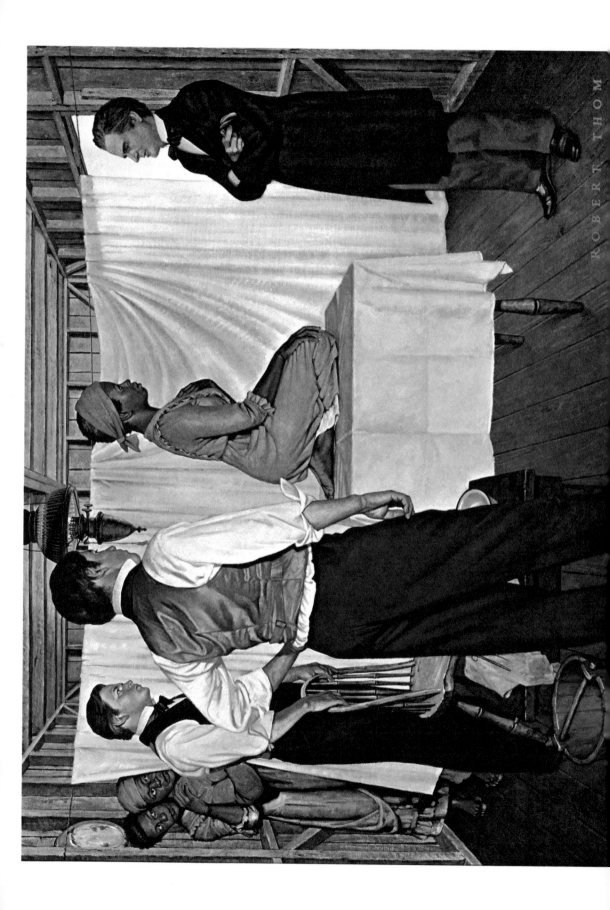

# J. MARION SIMS: GYNECOLOGIC SURGEON

Little did Dr. Marion Sims dream, in 1845, as he prepared to examine the slave girl, Lucy, that he was to become a woman's surgeon; or that his backyard structure in Montgomery, Alabama, would lead to opening of the nation's first Woman's Hospital, in New York, in 1855.

The idea that health problems peculiar to women deserve separate and distinct medical and surgical attention simply had not been conceived before the middle of the nineteenth century. Some physicians even refused to examine women or to treat them for other than ordinary afflictions. Their reasons ranged from realization of their own shortcomings to ludicrous pseudo modesty.

In maintaining this attitude, New World doctors of the early 1800's followed the practice of European physicians, to whom they looked for leadership in medicine. They were importers of ideas; seldom exporters. However, this trend began to change during the latter half of the century.

One who figured large in the change was James Marion Sims. During the early decades of the nineteenth century this name belonged only to a country boy growing up in North Carolina. In his youth and early manhood Marion showed little promise beyond the ordinary. Even after he graduated from Jefferson Medical College in Philadelphia in 1835 with an M.D. degree, nothing about him pointed to future greatness. But he was destined to launch a new medical specialty, gynecology.

Until 1845, Dr. Sims had taken little interest in women patients. Until June of that year, he had never encountered a case of vesicovaginal fistula; but during the next two months Dr. Sims was requested by the owners of three young female slaves, Anarcha, Betsy, and Lucy, who suffered from such fistulas, to do something to relieve them.

Three years of trial and error in trying to cure vesicovaginal fistula by surgery followed. Finally in 1849 Dr. Sims determined to use thin pure silver wires as sutures, securing them with pieces of lead. Anarcha became subject of the experiment; it was her thirtieth operation. The operation was successful; there was no infection about the silver wire sutures; the fistula was closed. In the next two weeks Lucy and Betsy were cured by similar operations.

Continued success in this type of surgery and in the treatment of other ailments of women patients led to the development of a new idea in Dr. Sims's mind: a special hospital for the care of women and for the performance of the operation at which he had become so adept. The idea took shape eventually in New York when Woman's Hospital was opened there May 4, 1855.

Dr. Marion Sims, to whom so many women owed lifelong debts of gratitude, indeed had a fruitful, inspiring career. Not only are the surgical feats he performed still outstanding; he led pioneers in gynecology to respectability and to recognition on a high plane. He invented new instruments to meet new requirements. He brought to medicine a new concept—hospitals devoted to the special needs of women. Equally important, he carried these bold, brilliant ideas, pioneered in America, to Europe and taught Old World physicians how to use them too.

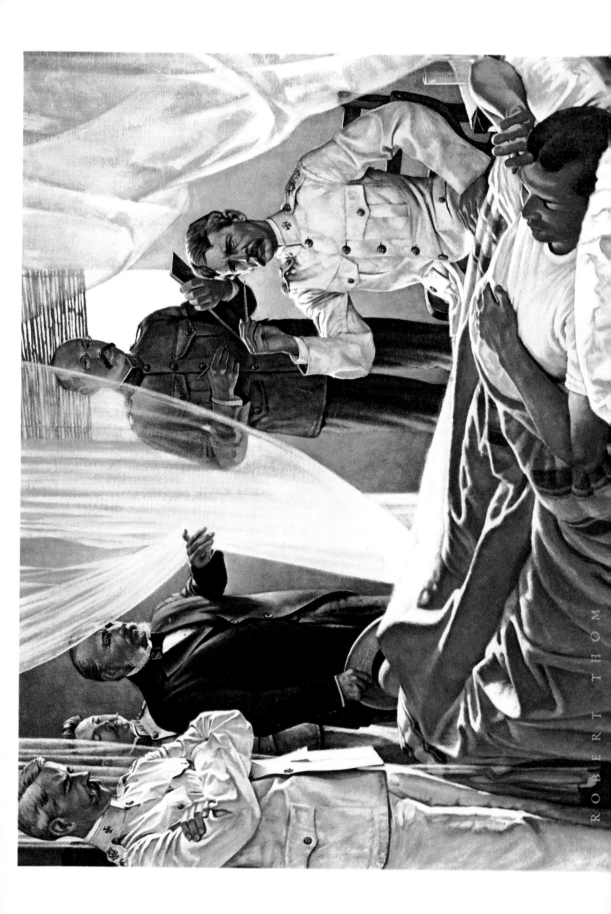

# THE CONQUEST OF YELLOW FEVER

Methods of preventing yellow fever developed from investigations which proved mosquitoes to be carriers of the virus, conducted in 1900 at Camp Lazear, Cuba, by a United States Army commission led by Dr. Walter Reed (seated), cooperating with Cuba's Dr. Carlos J. Finlay (in dark suit).

"I thank God that I did not accept anybody's opinion on this subject, but determined to put it to a thorough test with human beings in order to see what would happen. . . . Actual trial has proven that I was right."

Thus wrote Dr. Walter Reed, forty-nine-year-old surgeon with rank of major, United States Army, stationed at Columbia Barracks, Quemados, Cuba, on December 9, 1900, in a letter to his wife. Dr. Reed had been sent to Cuba by the Army's Surgeon General to head a commission to study yellow fever, and he was on the threshold of discovering how that dread disease was propagated.

Not far away, in Havana, undoubtedly another prayer of thanksgiving was in the mind of sixty-seven-year-old Dr. Carlos Juan Finlay, who at long last was witnessing men of science accepting and proving, beyond doubt, that his theories regarding transmission of yellow fever were correct.

Havana, Cuba, historically, had been a focus of yellow fever. After its occupation in 1898 in the course of the Spanish-American War, losses among United States troops became so great that Surgeon General Sternberg named a commission to go to Cuba to study the cause and transmission of yellow fever. Thus in 1900 persons most responsible for conquering the disease were brought together.

Major Walter Reed, chairman of the commission, and his group met Dr. Finlay, chairman of the cooperating Cuban Yellow Fever Commission and first man to point to the possible infective role of mosquitoes. Dr. Finlay, though firm in his convictions regarding a relationship between yellow fever and mosquitoes, had failed to gain the support of medical men. Reed and his associates now proceeded to clear up this controversial theory.

First man to be exposed in a daring experiment at Camp Lazear was Private John Kissinger. He with other brave volunteers had allowed themselves to be bitten by mosquitoes in a controlled situation that would definitely pinpoint the mosquito as the culprit if disease should occur. On December 8, 1900, Kissinger had the beginning of a well-defined attack of yellow fever.

Further experimental work of the United States commission, carried out largely by Dr. James Carroll, in charge of bacteriologic work of the commission, proved that the causative agent of yellow fever was not a bacterium, but a filterable virus which could be transmitted either by a mosquito bite or by injection of blood from a sick patient into the nonimmune subject. Translating the significance of this discovery into vigorous antimosquito measures, sanitation officers and squads were able to protect whole areas.

Thus was yellow fever, scourge of the centuries, conquered in half a century; that is, nearly conquered. It has virtually vanished from the world's major cities; but pools of the virus that defy eradication still lie deep in the world's tropical jungles.

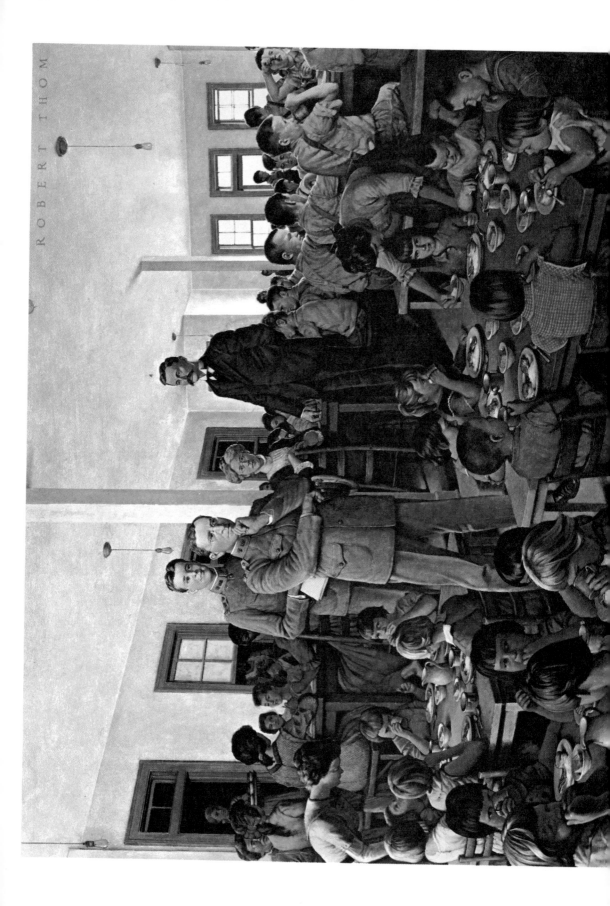

ROBERT THOM

# GOLDBERGER: DIETARY DEFICIENCY AND DISEASE

Dr. Joseph Goldberger (1874-1929), United States Public Health Surgeon, began studies of pellagra in 1914 near Jackson, Mississippi, in orphanages, asylums, and prisons. His research proved dietary deficiency the cause and directed other scientists toward discovery of vitamins.

When Dr. Joseph Goldberger, Surgeon, United States Public Health Service, and his assistant, Dr. C. H. Waring, began studies of pellagra at the Methodist and Baptist orphanages near Jackson, Mississippi, in 1914, they faced puzzling questions: Why were the adults, the older children, and the very young in these institutions free of the disease? Why, every year, did it strike children aged three to twelve? Dr. Goldberger ruled out infection and toxic foods as causes. With cooperation of Director J. R. Carter and House Mother "Miss Ida," the doctors added fresh meat, eggs, milk, oatmeal, peas, beans (foods commonly reserved for older people), and other vegetables to children's diets. Pellagra disappeared. By bold experiments Dr. Goldberger proved dietary deficiency the cause of pellagra and pointed the way toward discovery of health-sustaining vitamins.

Joseph Goldberger was born July 16, 1874, on a peasant farm near Giralt, Austria-Hungary (now a part of Czechoslovakia). When he was only seven years old, he came with his parents to America, the family settling in New York City. He chose medicine for his career; and after graduating from Bellevue Hospital Medical College, he entered the Public Health Service as an assistant surgeon and gained the reputation of being a "health detective."

Having scored successes in his study of measles, diphtheria, and other diseases, he was sent in 1914 by the surgeon general to the cotton country of the South to take over investigations of pellagra, a problem so widespread there that it was seriously affecting the economy.

Dr. Goldberger and his assistant set out to learn all they could about the disease. They went to cotton-mill towns; to the cotton fields; to the hills and valleys. They found hundreds of people afflicted with skin lesions, weakness, digestive upsets, diarrhea, and mental disturbances—typical signs of pellagra. But it was the suffering among the children in the two orphanages that challenged Dr. Goldberger most of all to discover the cause of the disease.

It was not long before the inquiring mind of the medical detective began to visualize patterns in the puzzle. Although the children's diet was adequate caloriewise, adults received considerably more meat and protein foods. The little children during their first two years received plenty of milk; but after that age, the children's diet was largely carbohydrate: corn bread, grits, cane syrup, and molasses.

To check his suspicions that the problem lay in a nutritional deficiency, Dr. Goldberger requested supplementary foods for the children in the age group most afflicted. Soon he noticed the signs of pellagra disappearing from the little faces. He launched similar studies at the Georgia State sanitarium and at the Mississippi State penitentiary. All tests proved pellagra could be prevented or cured by diet. His work prepared the way for other men to discover vitamin B and the part it plays in prevention of disease.

# Selective Atlas of
# Normal Anatomy

# Anatomy of the Heart

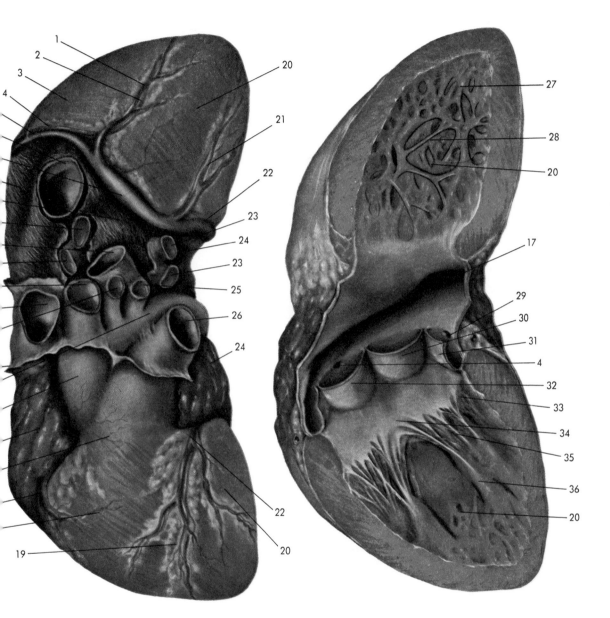

| | | |
|---|---|---|
| Middle cardiac vein | 13 Superior vena cava | 25 Left subclavian artery |
| Posterior descending branch of right coronary artery | 14 Left common carotid artery | 26 Left branch of pulmonary artery |
| Right ventricle | 15 Pericardium | 27 Trabeculae carneae |
| Right coronary artery | 16 Aortic arch | 28 Trabecula tendinea |
| Small cardiac vein | 17 Ascending aorta | 29 Left coronary artery |
| Inferior vena cava | 18 Conus arteriosus | 30 Posterior semilunar valve |
| Coronary sinus | 19 Anterior descending branch of left coronary artery | 31 Left semilunar valve |
| Right auricle | 20 Left ventricle | 32 Right semilunar valve |
| Left atrium | 21 Posterior vein of left ventricle | 33 Posterior cusp of mitral (bicuspid) valve |
| Right pulmonary vein | 22 Great cardiac vein | 34 Anterior cusp of mitral (bicuspid) valve |
| Right branch of pulmonary artery | 23 Left pulmonary vein | 35 Chordae tendineae |
| Innominate artery | 24 Left auricle | 36 Papillary muscle |

# Anatomy of the Stomach

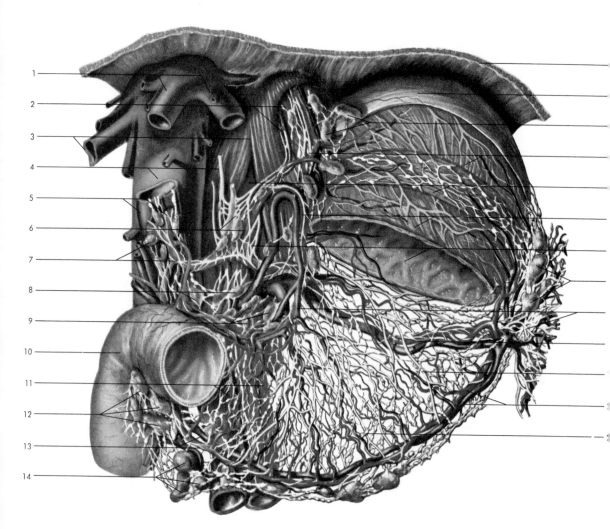

1 Middle and left hepatic veins
2 Right vagus nerve and esophagus
3 Right hepatic vein and crura of diaphragm
4 Inferior vena cava and greater splanchnic nerve
5 Portal vein and hepatic artery
6 Celiac plexus and celiac artery
7 Hepatic lymph node and hepatic rami of vagus nerve
8 Gastroduodenal artery and suprapyloric lymph nodes

9 Superior gastric lymph nodes
10 Duodenum
11 Superior mesenteric artery and vein
12 Subpyloric lymph nodes
13 Right gastroepiploic artery and vein
14 Inferior gastric lymph nodes
15 Diaphragm
16 Serosa
17 Paracardial lymph nodes
18 Left vagus nerve and longitudinal muscular layer

19 Abdominal aorta and circular muscular layer
20 Left gastric artery and oblique muscular layer
21 Celiac rami of vagus nerve and gastric mucosa
22 Splenic lymph nodes
23 Left gastric (coronary) vein and splenic rami of vagus nerve
24 Splenic artery and vein
25 Gastric rami of vagus nerve
26 Left gastroepiploic artery and vein
27 Gastric lymphatic plexus

## ABDOMINAL PORTION

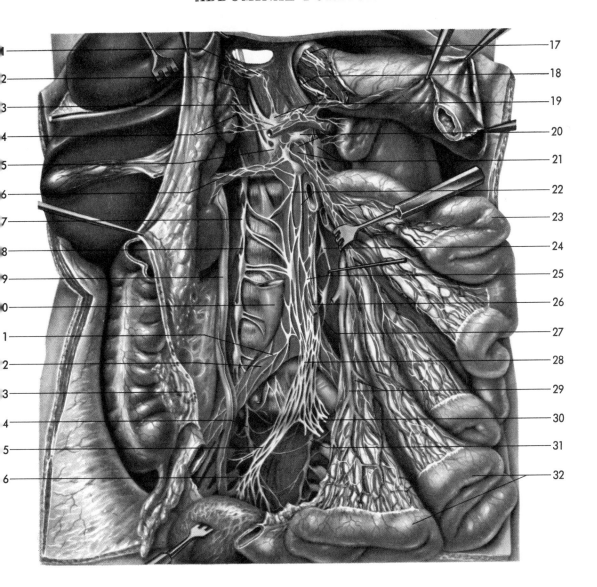

1 Phrenic ganglion and plexus
2 Greater splanchnic nerve
3 Lesser splanchnic nerve
4 Suprarenal plexus
5 Aorticorenal ganglion
6 Right renal artery and plexus
7 Right lumbar sympathetic ganglion
8 Right sympathetic trunk
9 Ureter
10 Vena cava
11 Iliac plexus

12 Right common iliac artery
13 Mesocolon (cut)
14 Right sacral sympathetic ganglion
15 Right pelvic plexus
16 Pudendal plexus
17 Left vagus nerve
18 Right vagus nerve
19 Celiac plexus and right celiac ganglion
20 Superior mesenteric ganglion and plexus
21 Left celiac ganglion; superior mesenteric artery

22 Abdominal aortic plexus
23 Jejunum
24 Left lumbar sympathetic ganglion
25 Inferior mesenteric ganglion
26 Inferior mesenteric plexus
27 Left sympathetic trunk
28 Hypogastric plexus
29 Branches of superior mesenteric artery and vein
30 Left pelvic plexus
31 Left sacral sympathetic ganglion
32 Ileum

# The Sympathetic Nervous System

## CEPHALIC, CERVICAL AND THORACIC PORTIONS

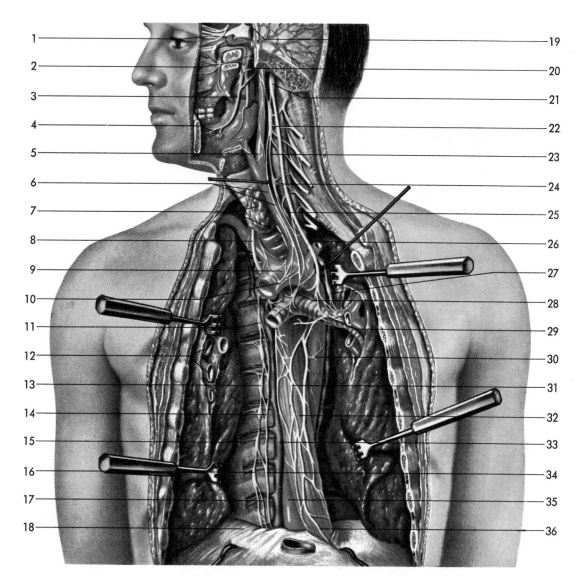

1 Ciliary ganglion
2 Sphenopalatine ganglion
3 Lingual nerve
4 Submandibular ganglion
5 Internal carotid artery
6 Common carotid artery; superior cardiac nerve
7 Thyroid gland; recurrent laryngeal nerve
8 Right vagus nerve
9 Aortic arch
10 Superficial cardiac plexus
11 Fifth thoracic sympathetic ganglion
12 Pulmonary artery and vein
13 Seventh thoracic sympathetic ganglion
14 Greater splanchnic nerve
15 Intercostal artery, vein and nerve
16 Tenth thoracic sympathetic ganglion
17 Lesser splanchnic nerve
18 Diaphragm
19 Trigeminal nerve
20 Otic ganglion
21 Nodose ganglion
22 Superior cervical sympathetic ganglion
23 Cervical sympathetic trunk
24 Middle cervical sympathetic ganglion
25 Inferior cervical sympathetic ganglio
26 Left vagus nerve
27 Fourth thoracic sympathetic ganglio
28 Cardiac ganglion
29 Anterior pulmonary plexus
30 Aortic plexus
31 Esophageal plexus
32 Esophagus
33 Azygos vein
34 Splanchnic ganglion
35 Aorta
36 Anterior gastric cord of vagus

# The Coronary Arteries

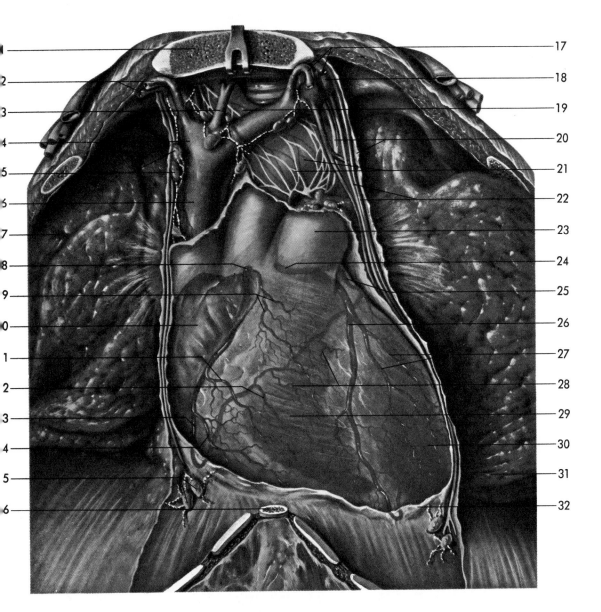

1 Manubrium
2 Right internal mammary artery and vein
3 Thyreoidea ima vein
4 Right brachiocephalic vein
5 Anterior superior mediastinal lymph nodes
6 Superior vena cava
7 Right lung
8 Right coronary artery
9 Preventricular arteries
10 Right atrium
11 Lateral branch of right coronary artery

12 Posterior descending branch of right circumflex artery
13 Right circumflex artery
14 Right marginal artery
15 Anterior inferior mediastinal lymph nodes
16 Xiphoid process
17 Left internal mammary artery and vein
18 Left brachiocephalic vein
19 Brachiocephalic trunk
20 Vagus nerve; mediastinal pleura (Cut)
21 Superficial cardiac plexus; arch of aorta

22 Pericardiacophrenic artery; phrenic nerve
23 Pulmonary artery
24 Left coronary artery
25 Left circumflex artery
26 Anterior descending branch of left coronary artery
27 Left marginal arteries
28 Left ventricular branches
29 Right ventricle
30 Left ventricle
31 Left lung
32 Pericardium (cut)

# Anatomy of the Ear

## FRONTAL SECTION SHOWING COMPONENT PARTS OF THE HUMAN EAR

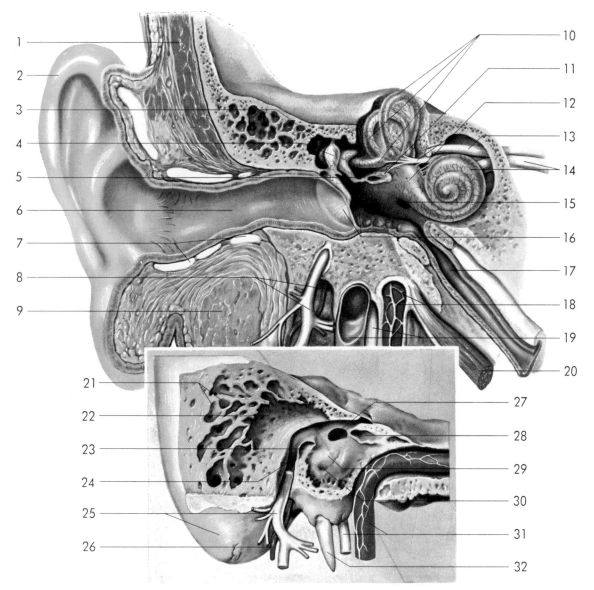

## SECTION THROUGH RIGHT TEMPORAL BONE SHOWING RELATIONSHIP BETWEEN MASTOID CELLS AND TYMPANIC CAVITY

1 Temporal muscle
2 Helix
3 Epitympanic recess
4 Malleus
5 Incus
6 External acoustic meatus
7 Cartilaginous part of external acoustic meatus
8 Facial nerve and stylomastoid artery
9 Parotid gland
10 Semicircular canals
11 Stapes
12 Vestibule and vestibular nerve

13 Facial nerve
14 Cochlea and cochlear nerve
15 Cochlear (round) window
16 Tympanic membrane and tympanic cavity
17 Auditory (Eustachian) tube
18 Internal carotid artery and sympathetic nerve plexus
19 Glossopharyngeal nerve and internal jugular vein
20 Levator veli palatini muscle
21 Mastoid cells
22 Tympanic antrum

23 Cavity of the pyramidal eminence for the stapedius
24 Facial canal
25 Facial nerve and mastoid process
26 Stylomastoid artery
27 Vestibular (oval) window
28 Cochleariform process
29 Promontory
30 Cochlear fenestra
31 Internal carotid artery and glossopharyngeal nerve
32 Styloid process

# VOLUME 3
New Edition

## You and Your Health

## More Diseases
## First Aid
## Emergencies

## In three volumes, illustrated

Harold Shryock, M.A., M.D., and
Mervyn G. Hardinge, M.D.,
Dr.P.H., Ph.D.
In Collaboration With 28 Leading Medical Specialists

Published jointly by

**PACIFIC PRESS PUBLISHING ASSOCIATION**
Boise, ID 83707
Oshawa, Ontario, Canada

**REVIEW AND HERALD PUBLISHING ASSOCIATION**
Washington, DC 20039-0555
Hagerstown, MD 21740

ISBN 0-8163-0535-8

You and Your Health
Volume 3
More Diseases
First Aid
Emergencies

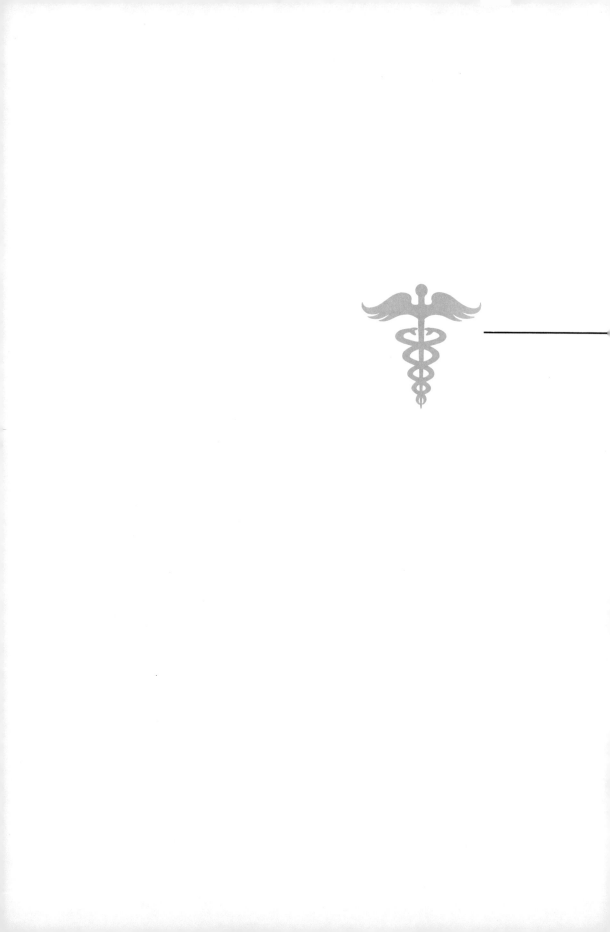

# SECTION III

# Cancer

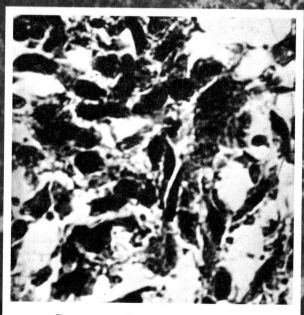
**Cancer—spoiler of pretty pictures.**

# Characteristics of Cancer

Cancer is the second most common cause of death in the United States, being exceeded only by diseases of the heart. In two years cancer kills more Americans than the total number killed in four recent wars: World War I, World War II, the Korean conflict, and the Vietnam engagement. Each year cancer kills about seven times the number of Americans killed in automobile accidents.

For one recent year the estimated number of new cases of cancer in the United States totaled 1,260,000, of which almost one third were cancer of the skin. For this same year deaths from cancer came to an estimated 420,000, a number approximately equal to the population of Atlanta, Georgia. Cancer of the lung accounts for the largest number of cancer deaths among men, and cancer of the breast among women. Present trends indicate, however, that lung cancer will also soon top the list for women.

Cancer is a tragic disease, not only because of the large number of deaths, but because of its high toll of human agony and suffering. The cancer victim who has received the best treatment

that medical science can provide still continues in a state of uncertainty for weeks, and perhaps months. He is haunted by the knowledge that the results of cancer treatment are commonly given in terms of five-year survival rates. He wonders whether he will be alive at the end of five years and, if so, what then?

### What Is Cancer?

A cancer is a kind of tumor that threatens life. So to understand the full meaning of the term *cancer* we must first explore the uses of the word *tumor*.

In its broad sense, a tumor means an abnormal enlargement of some part of the body. As usually used, the word refers to a mass of tissue composed of unusual cells that have multiplied more than they normally should, that are not a part of the body's normal design, and that serve no useful purpose. In this sense, the medical scientist prefers the term *neoplasm* (new growth) to the word *tumor*.

In the normal course of its development and growth, the human body maintains precise control over the

173

## LEADING CAUSES OF DEATH IN THE UNITED STATES

| Rank | Cause of Death | Number of Deaths | Percent of Total Deaths | Rank | Cause of Death | Number of Deaths | Percent of Total Deaths |
|---|---|---|---|---|---|---|---|
| | All Causes | 1,927,788 | 100.0 | 8. | Cirrhosis of Liver | 30,066 | 1. |
| | | | | 9. | Arteriosclerosis | 28,940 | 1. |
| 1. | Heart Diseases | 729,510 | 37.8 | 10. | Suicide | 27,294 | 1. |
| 2. | Cancer | 396,922 | 20.6 | | | | |
| 3. | Cerebrovascular | | | 11. | Diseases of Infancy | 22,033 | 1. |
| | diseases (Stroke) | 175,629 | 9.1 | 12. | Homicide | 20,432 | 1. |
| 4. | Accidents | 105,561 | 5.5 | 13. | Aortic Aneurysm | 14,028 | 0. |
| 5. | Pneumonia & Influenza | 58,319 | 3.0 | 14. | Congenital Anomalies | 12,968 | 0. |
| | | | | 15. | Pulmonary Infarction | 10,941 | 0. |
| 6. | Chronic Obstructive | | | | | | |
| | Lung Disease | 50,488 | 2.6 | | Other & Ill-defined | 210,606 | 10. |
| 7. | Diabetes Mellitus | 33,841 | 1.8 | | | | |

Source: American Cancer Society, Ca—A Cancer Journal for Clinicians, Jan/Feb 1983.

characteristics of the cells that compose its tissues. This control is mediated through the mysterious DNA molecules found in the nucleus of each one of the body's cells (see chapter 5, volume 2). The DNA molecules are "coded" to regulate the growth characteristics and activities of their respective cells, thus enabling them to work in cooperation with other cells.

As the body grows, beginning at conception and continuing to adulthood, the number of cells increases tremendously. This increase is carefully controlled so that only the proper number of each kind of cell is produced. But a developing neoplasm (tumor) is composed of cells which have multiplied irrespective of the body's normal checks and balances.

Tumors are subdivided into two large classes: benign and malignant. In the benign tumors the cells remain isolated from the surrounding tissues and grow within their own capsule. The word *benign* implies that this kind of tumor is harmless. But it does occupy space, and it therefore may cause trouble by exerting pressure on surrounding tissues. A fatty tumor which develops under the skin and which may cause a bump on the body's surface belongs to this benign class.

Malignant tumors are composed of cells so far out of control that they continue to multiply and invade the surrounding tissues. It is such a malignant tumor that is properly called a cancer. As a malignant tumor grows, it sends its processes like tentacles in many directions. As it invades other tissues, it often destroys them, usually by interfering with their supply of blood. Such destruction of the surrounding tissues may cause bleeding and ulceration.

The worst feature of malignant tumors (cancers) is that as their cells multiply and the tumor invades the surrounding tissues, small groups of these wild-growing cells may spread to other parts of the body. The cells may be carried by the bloodstream or the lymphatics, or they may adhere to the lining of body cavities. The new colony of wild cells will establish itself and develop a secondary tumor very much like the original one. The scientist speaks of this process of migration as metastasis. Often the metastatic tumors endanger the patient's life even more than the original tumor.

Most malignant tumors grow for a while at their site of origin before colonies of cells break away and move to some other region. From this observation we understand how important it is to treat a cancer early in the course of its development, before metastasis has taken place.

The specialty of medical science

# Manifestations of Cancer

In this chapter we list, in alphabetical order, the various parts of the body in which cancer may occur and describe its characteristics in these various locations.

## BILE DUCTS

The bile ducts may become involved either with cancer within the ducts or with cancer in neighboring structures. The earliest symptom is usually jaundice (manifested by a yellowing of the whites of the eyes and of the skin), an abnormality caused by obstruction to the flow of bile. Surgical treatment of cancer in this location is difficult, partly because of no alternate route for the flow of bile and partly because the cancer is usually advanced before the diagnosis is made.

## BLADDER (URINARY BLADDER)

Exposure to certain chemicals such as naphthalenes, aniline dyes, or benzidines predisposes to cancer of the bladder. These substances may be taken into the body by various routes but are eventually eliminated through the urinary system and thus appear in the urine as it is stored in the bladder. Cancer of the bladder often develops as a consequence of cigarette smoking because certain irritating substances in tobacco smoke are eliminated from the body through the urinary system.

The usual earliest sign of cancer of the bladder is blood in the urine (hematuria), often accompanied by pain. Cancer is not the only cause of blood in the urine, but whenever this symptom occurs, it should prompt examination of the urinary system to determine the cause of the bleeding.

Treatment of cancer of the bladder by surgery or by a combination of surgery and irradiation is quite successful when the cancer is detected and treated in its early stages.

## BLOOD

The disease leukemia, in which the tissues which form blood cells become involved, is classed as a cancer of the blood-forming tissues. See the discussion of leukemia in chapter 10, volume 2.

## BONE

Cancer of the bone may originate within the bone itself, it may have spread to the bone from cancer in adjacent structures, or it may develop secondarily when a colony of cancer cells is carried by the blood from a cancer in some other part of the body (by metastasis). Cancer of the bone typically

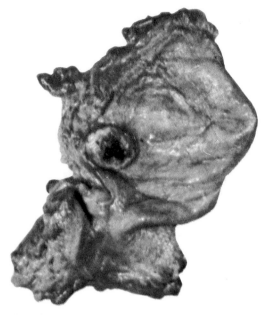

**Cancer of the bladder.**

causes considerable local pain and also a weakening of the bone so that it fractures easily (pathologic fracture). The treatment of cancer of the bone is difficult and may require radical surgery, irradiation therapy, or chemotherapy.

## BRAIN

The largest number of cases of cancer of the brain occur during childhood. Of all cases of childhood cancer, an estimated 19 percent involve the brain and/or other parts of the central nervous system.

Many cancers of the brain are said to be primary because they originate right in the brain substance. Others are classed as secondary or metastatic because a colony of cancer cells has migrated to the brain from a cancer in some other part of the body—most commonly from the lung or the breast.

A cancer developing within the brain is usually in the nature of a tumor that occupies more space than the normal tissue. Inasmuch as the brain is enclosed by the bony skull, a developing brain tumor typically produces abnormal pressure within the skull, which ac-

counts for many of the symptoms of brain cancer. This increased pressure affects everything within the skull, not just the area where the cancer is developing. Therefore, many of the symptoms do not give an accurate clue to the location of the cancer.

The most common symptom of cancer within the skull is headache, mild and intermittent at first, but becoming more severe and persistent. Then nausea and vomiting usually develop, along with drowsiness. The mental changes may include apathy, irritability, depression, and disturbances of consciousness. In about 50 percent of cases convulsive seizures develop at one time or another. A tumor in the area of the pituitary gland (at the base of the brain) usually produces significant disturbances in vision. In another area, toward the back of the brain, a developing tumor will cause disturbances of hearing and of equilibrium.

The patient with symptoms as above should be placed under the care of a physician who specializes in neurology or in brain surgery. Of the several tests and examinations that may be used to determine whether a brain cancer is present, the newer method of brain scan (computed axial tomography) is probably the most useful and accurate. It involves a sophisticated method of examination by X ray.

As with cancers in other locations, so with those of the brain: the earlier the diagnosis and treatment, the better the prospect for the patient's recovery. The specialty of brain surgery has made remarkable progress during recent years, and the lives of many patients with brain cancer can be spared by surgical removal of the involved area of the brain. In some cases, further treatment by irradiation is helpful.

## BREAST

The breast is the most common site of cancer in women, there being about 110,000 new cases a year in the United States and more than 37,000 deaths per year (data from the American Cancer Society, 1981).

190

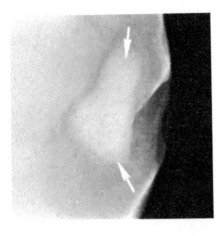

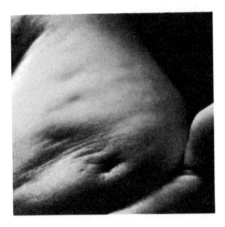

Top: X ray of axillary lymph nodes. A proven case of carcinoma of the breast with axillary metastases. Center: Adenocarcinoma, left breast. Below: Cancer of the breast, late stages of development.

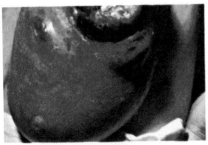

PUBLIC HEALTH SERVICE AUDIOVISUAL FACILITY

Cancer of the breast is treacherous because it tends to spread early to distant parts of the body. When breast cancer is detected before colonies of cancer cells have migrated to other areas, treatment by surgery and irradiation is quite successful.

Progress during recent years in reducing the mortality rate from cancer of the breast stems largely from early detection and adequate treatment. Women are becoming aware of the tragic outcome of a lump in the breast. By reporting this finding at once to her physician, a woman can receive the benefits of early treatment.

Only about one lump in five discovered in the breast proves to be caused by cancer. But this does not mean that a lump may be safely ignored, for the hazard of delay is so great that any lump discovered in the breast should be reported promptly.

In many instances the physician cannot determine by a simple examination whether a lump in the breast is cancerous or benign. So he removes a small portion of the tissue and arranges for a microscopic examination by a pathologist. If this biopsy specimen proves benign, the surgeon then performs a simple surgery to remove the lump. If, however, the biopsy examination indicates a beginning cancer, the entire breast should be removed, together with any lymph nodes in the axilla (armpit) that seem to have been already affected. This is the so-called modified radical surgical procedure for breast cancer, which spares the muscles located beneath the breast. This procedure may be followed by irradiation. If it appears that the cancer has already spread to other parts of the body by metastasis, the physician will determine the appropriate use of chemotherapy, irradiation, and surgery.

A lump in the breast may develop quickly without attracting particular attention. It may develop between the times of the periodic checkups at the doctor's office. So it is now advocated that women learn the method of self-examination of the breast, as here illus-

**191**

# Breast Self-examination

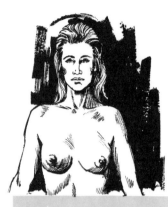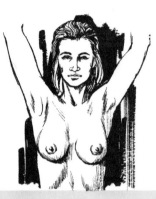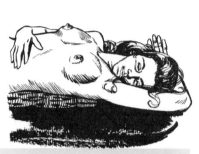

1. Examination of breasts before a mirror for symmetry in size and shape, noting any puckering of skin or retraction of nipple.

2. Arms raised over head, again studying breasts in the mirror for the same signs.

3. Reclining on bed with flat pillow or folded bath towel under shoulder on same side as breast to be examined.

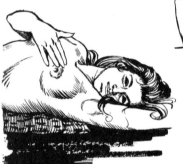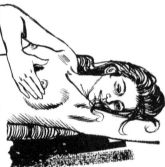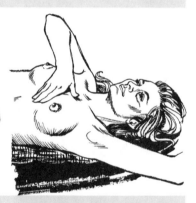

4. To examine inner half of the breast, arm is raised. Beginning at breastbone and working out, inner half of breast is palpated.

5. The area over and around the nipple is carefully palpated with flats of the fingers.

6. Continuing thus to palpate, examination of lower inner half of the breast is completed.

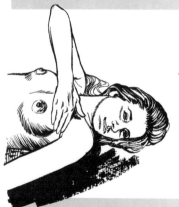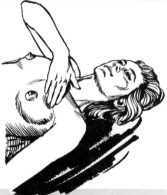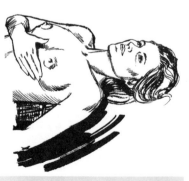

7. With arm down at side, palpation continues with examination of tissues extending to armpits.

8. The upper outer quadrant of the breast is examined with the flat part of the fingers.

9. The lower outer quadrant of the breast is likewise examined in successive stages.

# Dietary
# Problems

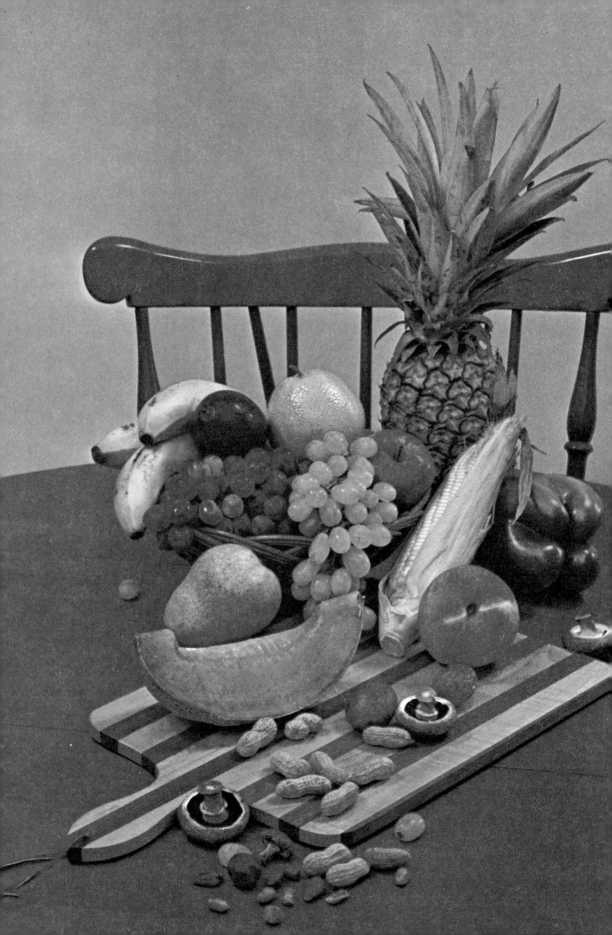

# Deficiency Diseases

The deficiency diseases are caused by a shortage in the diet of certain food constituents even when the total amount of food may be adequate.

This chapter is concerned mostly with the body's need for vitamins, minerals, and proteins, and with the consequences when certain of these are in short supply. Consideration is also given to the advisability, and even to the possible hazards, of taking vitamins and minerals as medications or as dietary supplements.

## A. Avitaminoses

Illnesses that stem from a shortage of certain vitamins are collectively called the avitaminoses—the prefix *a* indicating "a lack of."

### VITAMIN A DEFICIENCY

A mild deficiency of vitamin A tends to produce roughness and dryness of the skin. Another common symptom is night blindness, in which the ability to see in dim light is reduced. A great degree of deficiency causes damage to the epithelial tissues of the body, which then become more susceptible to infection. In later stages, severe infections of the mouth, the genitourinary tract, the respiratory organs, and the eyes may occur. The eye infection often develops into, or in connection with, a serious condition called xerophthalmia, which may lead to blindness.

Some evidence suggests that a lack of vitamin A predisposes to cancer. On the other hand, there has been considerable research into the use of retinoids (both natural and synthetic forms of vitamin A) in the treatment of various types of cancer, with promising results.

Adequate amounts of vitamin A are contained in the usual average American diet. This vitamin is especially abundant in such foods as carrots, sweet potatoes, apricots, orange squash, cheese, and milk.

The recommended daily allowance (RDA) for vitamin A varies from about 1500 international units for infants to about 5000 international units for adults. Danger lurks in taking large supplements of vitamin A. It has been demonstrated that doses of 50,000 international units or more per day continued for weeks or months produce such symptoms as loss of appetite, blurred vision, cracking of the skin, headaches, diarrhea, and nausea.

#### Care and Treatment

**Treatment for such conditions as night blindness or other symptoms of mild deficiency of vitamin A consists of the administration of 25,000 international units of vitamin A each day for a period of one or two weeks. In serious deficiencies such as**

xerophthalmia, the physician may prescribe daily injections of the water-dispersible form of vitamin A in doses up to 100,000 international units continued for a few days, followed by smaller doses by mouth over a period of several weeks.

## VITAMIN B DEFICIENCIES

The B group of vitamins includes these: (1) thiamine (vitamin $B_1$), (2) riboflavin (vitamin $B_2$), (3) niacin or nicotinic acid, (4) vitamin $B_{12}$, (5) folic acid, and (6) vitamin $B_6$ (pyridoxine). We consider the deficiencies of each of these separately.

1. *Thiamine (Vitamin $B_1$ Deficiency)*. The disease beriberi is caused by thiamine deficiency. It is characterized by an inflammation and degeneration of nerve trunks, with resulting disturbances of both motion and sensation. The patient loses his appetite and becomes weak, especially in the legs. The nerves controlling the action of the heart may be affected, and heart failure and sudden death may result.

Beriberi occurs most frequently among people whose diet consists mostly of polished rice, but anybody who lives chiefly on highly refined starchy or sugary foods may get it. It may develop in infants, especially those nursed by mothers who have the disease.

If the disease is not far advanced, correction of diet usually will bring about rapid and complete recovery. If the neuritis has continued until the nerve trunks have degenerated, however, normal motion, sensation, and heart action may never be restored.

Wernicke's encephalopathy is another condition caused by a deficiency of thiamine. It occurs most commonly among heavy users of alcohol. For a further discussion of Wernicke's encephalopathy, see chapter 4 in this volume.

Thiamine deficiency is prevented by a diet which includes whole cereals (unrefined), nuts, milk and milk products, fruits, and vegetables. Meat also contains a moderate amount of thiamine.

### Care and Treatment

A severe case of beriberi constitutes a medical emergency. The treatment should start with one injection (into a muscle) of 60 mg. of thiamine. Thereafter for one to two weeks the patient should receive thiamine by mouth in three or four doses per day to make a daily total of 25 mgs. From then on, the dose of thiamine taken by mouth should be reduced to 2.5 mg. per day.

2. *Riboflavin (Vitamin $B_2$) Deficiency*. Riboflavin deficiency develops gradually, the early evidence being a development of fissures (cracking) at the corners of the mouth and in the lips. The tongue becomes unnaturally smooth and has an unnatural red color. In children, riboflavin deficiency impedes normal growth. Also the eyes are commonly affected, with the cornea becoming opaque in extreme cases.

Prevention of riboflavin deficiency requires plenty of milk in the diet, milk being the outstanding dietary source of riboflavin. This vitamin is also contained, however, in eggs, green vegetables, and meat.

### Care and Treatment

Three to 10 mg. of riboflavin should be given by mouth three times each day until the patient shows improvement. Then the dose can be reduced to 1 mg. three times a day until recovery is complete.

3. *Niacin (Nicotinic Acid) Deficiency*. Beginning in the eighteenth century and continuing through the nineteenth, there appeared a disease known as pellagra, characterized by three D's: dermatitis, diarrhea, and dementia. It became prevalent in northern Spain and Italy, and, eventually, in southern United States. It often affected several members of the same family, particularly families whose diet was meager. In 1927 it was discovered that pellagra is the result of a deficiency

# Allergies and Infections

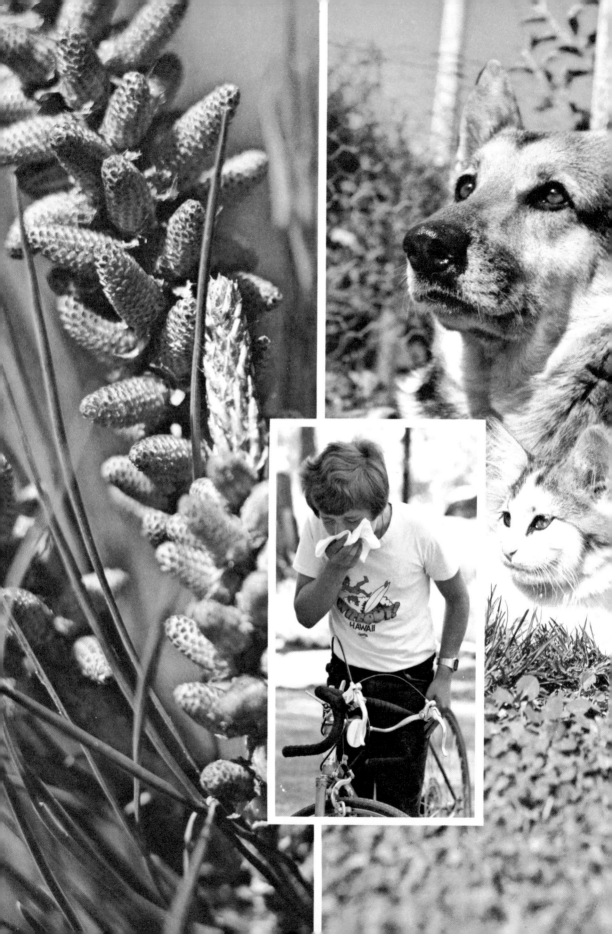

Section V

*CHAPTER* 14

# *Allergic Manifestations*

It is not intended that this chapter will add significantly to our list of diseases. It is expected, rather, that it will improve the reader's understanding of the causes of some of the diseases described in other parts of the book.

In the broad sense, allergy is the body's response to the presence of some aggravating agent called an allergen. Individuals react differently in their responses to allergens; therefore some people are said to be more allergic than others.

It used to be assumed that all allergens were protein substances, and it was common to speak of "protein sensitivity," by which was meant that a given protein substance would cause certain tissues to react abnormally. It is now understood that some allergens are carbohydrates, and at least a few are chemically related to the fats. Regardless of their chemical nature, all allergens have one thing in common— they stimulate a sensitive individual to react by producing antibodies.

The mechanism by which tissues react unfavorably to the presence of an allergen is bound up with the body's intricate chemical processes, such as enzyme reactions, and is even related to the processes by which immunity is developed. Becoming immune to a cer-

tain germ whose products have served as an allergen is one form of response which could be thought of as allergy but is best termed immunity. When the antibodies which a certain allergen produces are fixed to a group of the body's cells rather than remaining free in the bloodstream, then these cells on which the antibodies are located may be unfavorably affected when exposed to this specific allergen.

### Kinds of Allergens

1. Some allergens enter the body by being inhaled. These include pollens; dusts; vapors, such as tobacco smoke; emanations from epithelium, such as dandruff; and strong odors, such as perfumes.

2. Certain foods provoke an allergic response in persons who may be sensitive. These include wheat, milk, chocolate, eggs, strawberries, nuts, pork, and fish.

3. Some persons become sensitive to drugs or biological agents. These substances, then, can serve as allergens.

4. Certain germs may function as allergens so that the symptoms produced when these germs invade a person's tissues are the direct result of the allergic response and are not caused, primarily,

235

by tissue injury through direct contact with the germs.

5. Some allergens cause the allergic response through a mere contact with the skin or the mucous membranes of a sensitive person. These include products from plants such as poison oak and poison ivy, and certain dyes, metals, plastics, furs, leathers, rubber products, cosmetics, and chemicals such as insecticides.

6. Even physical agents such as heat, cold, light, and pressure occasionally awaken a response similar to an allergy. Many a sufferer from hay fever has noticed that he begins to sneeze when he steps into bright sunlight. This can be either a triggering of the allergy or a vasomotor response due to sensitive membranes and thus not a true allergy.

### Preventing the Allergic Response

In general, the allergic response may be prevented or its symptoms modified in four ways:

A. *Avoiding the Allergen.* The simplest way to prevent the allergic response is to prevent the allergens to which a person is sensitive from entering his body. Sufferers from hay fever can often prevent their attacks by staying indoors during the time of year when the plants bloom that produce the pollens to which they are sensitive. If these plants are limited to a certain locality, the sufferers can avoid symptoms by staying away from this locality. Allergy to a drug can be avoided by not using the drug. Allergy to some specific food may be handled by excluding this food from the diet. Persons sensitive to a particular dust may benefit by wearing a filtering mask. Airconditioning systems with good filters often bring relief to victims of hay fever and asthma.

B. *Desensitization.* Just as it is possible to make a person immune to snake venom by injecting gradually increasing doses of this venom into his tissues, so it is possible to build up a person's tolerance to some allergens by a carefully controlled program of administering gradually increasing doses of this allergen. Physicians can obtain preparations of the usual allergens from medical supply houses and can inject these into a sensitive patient, beginning with very small doses and building up gradually week by week, until the patient's tolerance has improved to the point where he will no longer develop symptoms when exposed to the allergen. This method has proved quite successful in bringing relief to many patients suffering from hay fever and to some suffering from types of asthma which result in large part from allergy. It may be necessary to administer doses of these preparations at regular intervals the year round in order to maintain the individual's tolerance to the offending substance.

C. *The Use of Antihistamines.* In most cases of allergy, histamine is one of the chemicals which the body's tissues liberate in response to the presence of an allergen. An antihistamine drug, which counteracts histamine, may relieve the allergic response in such cases. There are many varieties of antihistamine drugs, and it happens that one kind will benefit some allergic persons and another kind, others. It may be necessary to use the trial-and-error method to determine which form of antihistamine will bring the greatest benefit in a particular case. Some hay fever sufferers derive enough benefit from the use of antihistamines that they prefer using them to obtaining relief by the more time-consuming desensitization method.

Some hazard is involved in the use of antihistamine drugs, because in some cases these have the side effect of making a person sleepy. It is dangerous, therefore, for the person taking such drugs to drive a car lest his reactions have been slowed to the extent that his driving is unsafe.

D. *The Use of Hormones.* In cases of extremely serious allergic reactions,

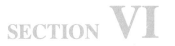

SECTION **VI**

**First Aid;
Poisoning;
Emergencies**

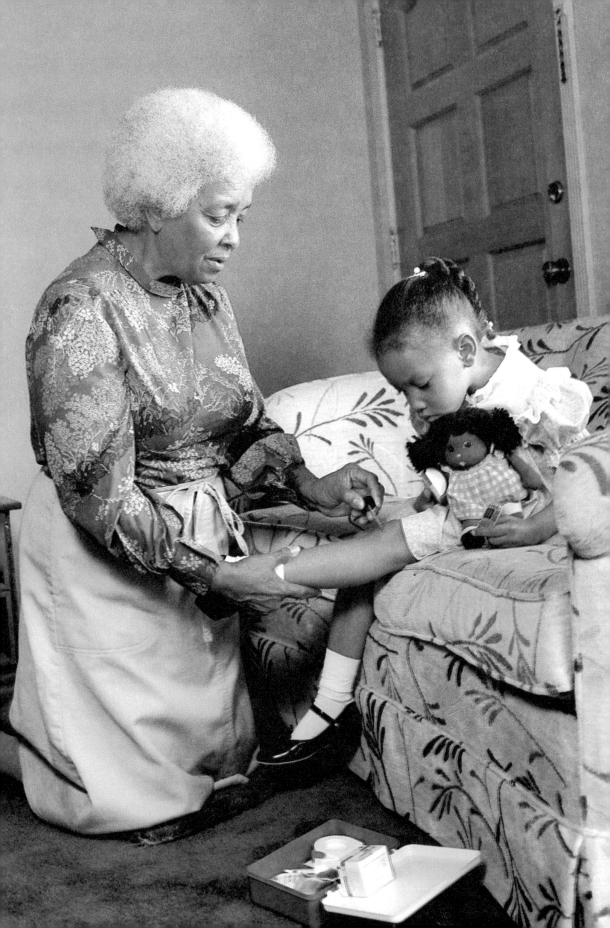

# First-aid Kits and Home Medicine Chests

The prevalence of accidents in and around the home and on highways makes first-aid kits a necessity in every household and in every car. Extensive experience indicates that a small transportable emergency kit for the home should contain at least the following articles, most of which can be purchased at the drugstore:

Box of adhesive bandages about 1 x 3 inches (2.5 x 7.5 cm.) in size.

Box of adhesive bandages half as wide as the above.

Sterile gauze squares, about 3 x 3 inches (7.5 x 7.5 cm.), preferably in individual packages—at least a dozen.

Pieces of sterile gauze about one yard (meter) square, in individual packages—at least three.

Triangular bandages—at least three.

Roller bandages, 1-inch (2.5 cm.) and 2-inch (5 cm.) widths.

Some approved variety of burn ointment.

Small bottle of aromatic spirits of ammonia.

Small bottle of antiseptic solution.

Scissors, medium size.

Wire or thin board splints—at least two long and two short.

The kit to be carried in the car need not include so many articles. The following are recommended:

One roll of 1-inch (2.5 cm.) width adhesive tape.

Six small adhesive bandages.

Six 3 x 3 inch (7.5 x 7.5 cm.) sterile gauze squares, packaged separately.

One yard square (meter) of bandaging material (muslin).

One tube of approved variety of burn ointment.

One small bottle of antiseptic.

Kits to be carried in the car should be kept in canvas rolls or metal containers. Those for the home may also be kept in metal cases or boxes. Avoid the tendency to keep articles for home first-aid use lying around in different drawers or piled on shelves. Places specified for these articles should not be used for anything else. The materials should be kept in good order in the case or box, arranged so that any desired article can be found without unpacking everything in the kit, and the separate packages should be wrapped in such a way that unused material will not be soiled by handling.

The bottle of aromatic spirits of ammonia should be replaced with a new one every year to ensure full strength always. Certain antiseptics also contain a volatile substance which makes periodic replacement of them likewise necessary, perhaps even every six months.

Various manufacturers put up special individual packages or kits, often of sizes and shapes convenient for packing into cases for first-aid use. Also these kits are packed so as to prevent contamination or spoilage, generally with printed directions for use on the outside of each package. If you are willing to spend a little more to obtain your first-aid supplies in such forms, you will probably feel repaid in the long run. Your druggist will doubtless be able to show you samples.

### Home Medicine Chests

In some homes, the first-aid kit and the home medicine cabinet are combined, but it is better to have a separate medicine cabinet, preferably in the bathroom. The ordinary small cabinet usually installed above the lavatory and kept more or less full of toilet articles will not serve the purpose adequately. Separate shelves out of reach of children, or preferably a separate cabinet equipped with a lock, should be built and kept solely for medicines and treatment supplies. The following is a suggested list of contents—sizes and measurement being given in both standard and metric units, which, however, in most cases are not precisely equivalent:

# Home Medicine Chest: Suggested Contents

Absorbent cotton, sterile—4 oz. or 100 gm.

Activated charcoal—4 oz. or 100 gm.

Adhesive tape, 1-inch (2.5 cm.) width—1 roll.

Antiseptic, one bottle.

Antiseptic soap.

Aromatic spirits of ammonia—2 oz. or 50 ml.

Aspirin tablets.

Baby oil.

Bedpan.

Boric acid ointment, 5 percent—2 oz. or 50 mg.

Calamine lotion—4 oz. or 100 ml.

Clinical thermometer, mouth style.

Earache drops—1 oz. or 25 ml.

Enema kit.

Epsom salts—1 pound or 500 mg.

Eucalyptus oil—2 oz. or 50 ml.

Gauze roller bandage, 1-inch (2.5 cm.)—1 roll.

Gauze roller bandage, 2-inch (5 cm.)—1 roll.

Glycerin—8 oz. or 200 ml.

Hot-water bottle.

Hydrogen peroxide, 8 oz. or 200 ml.

Ice bag.

Lysol, 4 oz. or 100 ml. (label as poison).

Medicine droppers—two.

Milk of magnesia—8 oz. or 200 ml.

Mineral oil—1 pint or 500 ml.

Mustard powder—4 oz. or 100 gm.

Nose drops.

Oil of cloves—$1/2$ oz. or 10 ml.

Petrolatum (vaseline)—4 oz. or 100 gm.

Potassium permanganate crystals—2 oz. or 50 gm.

Razor blades (stiff-backed).

Rubbing alcohol—1 pint or 500 ml.

Safety matches.

Safety pins, medium size—one dozen.

Scissors, medium size.

Syringe, soft rubber—2 oz. or 50 ml. size.

Syrup of ipecac—2 oz. or 50 ml.

Tylenol tablets.

Zinc oxide ointment—1 oz. or 25 gm.

Zinc stearate powder—2 oz. or 50 gm.

The list of items and the amounts given above are only general suggestions. There may be other articles or substances which your experience will prove necessary for your family. On the other hand, some in this list you may not require. You would be unwise to keep your medicine cabinet cluttered up with items or substances which you seldom use. The nearer you are to a drugstore and the more convenient it is for you to buy what you need, the fewer the articles you will need to keep readily on hand at home.

### Special Classes of Medicines

Certain home remedies which householders usually include in a medicine chest deserve special mention:

*Analgesics.* These are pain relievers, often more harmful than beneficial. Aspirin is probably the least harmful, but it is one especially to be kept out of the reach of children, as it constitutes the most common cause of child poisoning. Oil of cloves for tooth ache is another common analgesic.

*Antacids.* These are used to counter excess acid in the stomach. Magnesium carbonate, aluminum hydroxide, and magnesium trisilicate are the commonly used antacids and constitute the active ingredients of commercial preparations obtainable at drugstores. Baking soda (sodium bicarbonate), though often used as an antacid, is not recommended for this purpose.

*Antiseptics.* For superficial wounds which may become infected, present usage favors thorough cleansing with soap and water in preference to chemical antiseptics. However, many persons still feel more secure against infection if they apply an antiseptic preparation such as can be obtained from the drugstore. The reader may check with his pharmacist for a recommended brand. Also available commercially are disinfectants useful for decontaminating articles used in caring for wounds. Lysol solution is a well-known example. The householder or first-aid worker will of course recognize that these preparations are not to be administered internally.

*Cathartics.* A continuous use of cathartics entails the risk of developing the carthartic habit. But an occasional dose of Epsom salts or milk of magnesia for constipation will do little or no harm. However, *even the simplest cathartic may be hazardous if taken when a person has abdominal pain.* In case such pain is due to an inflamed appendix the use of a cathartic may dangerously aggravate the condition.

*Emetics.* These are substances that produce vomiting. To induce vomiting have the victim drink lukewarm water (plain or containing a little salt, baking soda, or soap) after which the first-aider places his finger in the victim's throat, causing him to gag and thus to vomit. If syrup of ipecac is available, it may be used as directed on page 334, PROCEDURE E, *To Induce Vomiting.*

*Hypnotics.* These are sleep producers. Their common or habitual use is recognized as harmful. They should be used only as prescribed by a physician.

*Stimulants.* In conditions such as poisoning, shock, or heat exhaustion the patient, if conscious, may be given a teaspoonful of aromatic spirits of ammonia in a glass of cool water. Also a drink of warm coffee may be given; however, for reasons stated elsewhere (see chapter 54, volume 1, pages 491-493), this beverage, like other stimulants, is not recommended for nonmedicinal use. A warm, strong coffee enema may be given to even an unconscious patient suffering from the above-mentioned conditions.

### Caution With Poisons

The home medicine cabinet may contain a few substances that are poisonous, including even "safe" preparations if taken in excess. Treatment for poisoning is outlined in the following chapter.

It is dangerous to take any substance the nature or identity of which is not absolutely clear. If bottles or packages lose their labels, the contents should be flushed down the toilet. Keep your medicine chest in good order; it could mean the saving of a life.

# *Poisonings*

## General Considerations

It is estimated that more than a million cases of poisoning occur each year in the United States, with about 6000 deaths. A large percentage of poisoning cases occur in children, and of these children, 80 percent are between the ages of 1 and 4. The most common cause of poisoning in children is the taking of many tablets of flavored, chewable baby aspirin.

Among adults, barbiturate medicines come first, with methyl alcohol (wood alcohol) and the various kinds of denatured alcohols coming second.

Even newborn babies are not immune. Boric acid solutions have been used accidentally as diluent in babies' formulas, causing a number of deaths.

Widespread knowledge of first-aid procedures, prompt and efficient action by physicians in general, and recent development in all major cities of poison-control centers have greatly reduced deaths from accidental poisoning. In view, however, of still high percentages of children involved in accidental poisonings, parents also must join hands in helping to prevent these accidents. Therefore the inclusion of vital information on this subject as a separate chapter in *You and Your Health.*

*Prevention Rather Than Cure.* One's conduct, particularly at home, is determined largely by habit. Habits of taking precautions and avoiding risks are life-saving in the long run, whereas habits of carelessness and attitudes of "It can't happen to me" form the prelude to misfortune. To prevent poisoning accidents, first, recognize the hazards and, second, adopt and enforce policies for the home and members of the family which remove the conditions under which such accidents can occur.

### How to Poison-proof Your Home

The American Medical Association provides the following list of seven precautions, which, when put into effect, will eliminate practically all danger of accidental poisoning:

1. Make sure to keep all drugs, poisonous substances, and household chemicals out of the reach of children. (Remember children can climb.)

2. Do not store nonedible products on shelves used for storing food.

3. Keep all poisonous substances in their original containers; don't transfer them to unlabeled containers.

4. When medicines are discarded, destroy them. Don't throw them where they may be reached by chil-

NOTE: The following section on first aid for poisoning conforms to the recommendations made at the Joint Symposium of the American Academy of Clinical Toxicology, the American Association of Poison Control Centers, and the Canadian Academy of Clinical Toxicology, held in 1976.

# POISONS

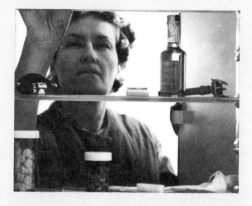

dren or pets. Flush them down the toilet.

5. When giving flavored or brightly colored medicine to children, always refer to it as medicine—never as candy.

6. Do not give or take medicine in the dark.

7. *Read labels* before using chemical products.

### Poison-proof Instructions for Specific Rooms

*The Kitchen.* More poisonings occur here than in any other room in the house—an estimated 34 percent. Poi-

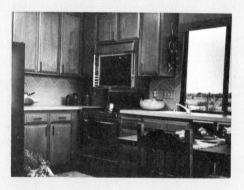

son-proof your kitchen, therefore, by keeping all dangerous household agents by themselves, separate from food, in their original containers and properly labeled, and out of reach of children.

*The Bedroom.* Here about 27 percent of all poisoning accidents take place. From what? Mothballs, cosmetics, cleaning agents stored in the closet, and from sleeping pills and other medicines placed on the night stand.

How to poison-proof the bedroom? Two simple directives to follow: (1) Keep all poisonous agents and medicines in their proper containers and stored in places inaccessible to children; and (2) keep medicines where they cannot be reached "conveniently" by a person too sleepy to be aware of what he is doing.

*The Bathroom.* This is the location for about 15 percent of all poisoning ac-

cidents. Poison-proof by keeping all medicines in a locked cupboard and placing the key well out of reach of children.

*The Living Room.* This is the locale of some 9 percent of all poisoning accidents. How can one poison-proof this room? Do not allow cosmetics, cleaning agents, and medicines to accumulate here, where they don't belong anyway.

*The Garage, Yard, and Basement.* Cans of petroleum products, solvents, pesticides, and those magic chemicals used around the car, house, and yard are kept here—substances which cause about 16 percent of all poisoning accidents.

Poison-proof by keeping all chemicals in plainly labeled containers and stored out of the reach of children. Many a child's life has been in danger because he mistook some household solvent in an unlabeled pop bottle as good to drink.

### General Symptoms of Poisoning

These are often confusingly similar to the symptoms of some of the infectious diseases and include loss of appetite, pain in the abdomen, a feeling of being sick at the stomach with a tendency to vomit, and diarrhea.

Also, a poison victim's skin may be cold, clammy, and blue-colored. There may be loss of consciousness and even convulsions.

# First Aid for Poisoning

**POISONS**

The outcome of a case of poisoning depends a great deal on the way it is handled by the first person who renders help—very often the mother of a child. Speed being the essence of success, the judgment of the first-aider is of prime importance.

## THE EMERGENCY CALL

Once poisoning is suspected, place an emergency call at once for a physician, the emergency squad of the fire department, or **the poison control center of your nearest city.** Preferably this call should be placed by a second responsible person so that the first-aider can devote all his time to the care of the patient. In placing the call, give as much information as possible: the patient's name, any clue as to the nature of the poison (such as the wording of the label on the container), the patient's symptoms, and the patient's exact present whereabouts. The person placing the call should ask for instructions on how to care for the patient until help arrives or while the patient is being taken to an emergency room.

### First Aid for Poisons
### Injected Through the Skin

This includes poisoning by snakebite or by the sting of an insect. For first-aid procedures see under *Bites* in this volume, pages 362-366, and under *Stings* in this volume, pages 413, 414.

### First Aid for
### Poisoning by Skin Contact

Contact with substances spilled on the skin may cause not only burns but systemic poisoning by absorption of the chemical through the skin. For first-aid procedures, see under *Burns—Burns Caused by Chemicals* on page 372 of this volume.

### First Aid for
### Poisoning by Inhalation

When the victim has breathed a poison gas (such as carbon monoxide), remove him from the room or area in which he has inhaled the gas and administer artificial respiration as necessary to keep him breathing. (See under *Respiratory Failure* in this volume,

**In any case of poisoning
CALL POISON CONTROL CENTER
in your area without delay.**

pages 407-409.) Call for trained help. If a tank of oxygen is available, waft a stream of the oxygen gas under the victim's nose so that he breathes it.

### First Aid for
### Poisoning by Mouth

Try to learn the nature of the poison or the medicine that has been swallowed. Give all such information to the doctor, the emergency squad, or the poison control center when making the emergency call previously mentioned. Save the container, if available, and any remaining portion of the poison or medicine. Save the stomach contents if and when the patient vomits. All of these items are to be examined by the doctor or the poison specialist who takes over the case.

The particular kind of first aid for a person who has swallowed a poison or taken an overdose of medicine depends on his present condition and on the kind of poison or medicine swallowed.

So there comes next a listing of the five general procedures, designated as A, B, C, D, and E, each adapted to a particular situation. The first-aider should check through these and choose the one that fits the case he is handling. If in doubt on which procedure to use, he can refer to the *Alphabetical Listing of Specific Poisons* which begins on page 335.

### General Procedures for
### Poisonings by Mouth

**PROCEDURE A.** *When the victim is unconscious.* Call for trained help. Administer artificial respiration as neces-

**POISONS**

sary to keep the patient breathing. (See under *Respiratory Failure* in this volume, pages 407-409.) Do not give fluids while the patient is unconscious. Do not force the unconscious patient to vomit; but if he does so spontaneously, turn his head so that the vomitus drains out of his mouth. Save the vomitus for later examination.

**PROCEDURE B.** *When the victim has swallowed a petroleum product* such as kerosene, gasoline, benzine, paint thinner, fuel oil, and naphtha. Call for trained help. Arrange to take the victim to a hospital as soon as possible because of the great danger of a serious type of pneumonia.

Remove any contaminated clothing and wash the underlying skin. Keep the victim quiet and warm. Use artificial respiration as necessary to keep the victim breathing. (See under *Respiratory Failure* in this volume, pages 407-409.) If a tank of oxygen is available, waft a stream of the oxygen gas under the victim's nose so that he breathes it. **Do not force the victim** to vomit except under a doctor's order and supervision. Give a glass of milk to drink so as to dilute the stomach contents. Give egg white or crushed banana by mouth to soothe the inflamed membranes.

**PROCEDURE C.** *When the victim has swallowed a corrosive poison* such as strong acid or alkali. Common examples are lye, caustic soda, drain and toilet-bowl cleaners, and electric dishwasher detergents in either solid or liquid form. There may or may not be burns on the lips and around the mouth. The severe damage occurs inside the mouth and in the lining of the esophagus.

Call at once for trained help. Plan for hospitalization. Dilute the caustic agent at once by giving the victim a drink of milk (or water if milk is not at hand). Remove any contaminated clothing and wash the underlying skin. Do not try to make the victim vomit. Irritations of the lining membranes may be soothed by having the patient swallow cream or egg white. Keep the victim quiet and warm. Use cracked ice to relieve thirst.

**PROCEDURE D.** *When the victim is having convulsions.* Do not try to prevent the patient's movements but do what is necessary to keep him from injuring himself. (See *Convulsions* in this volume, page 380.) Do not give fluids by mouth. Do not force the patient to vomit; but if he vomits spontaneously, turn his head so that the material drains from his mouth.

**PROCEDURE E.** *When the victim is conscious, is NOT having convulsions, and has NOT swallowed a petroleum product or a corrosive poison.* Three principles are followed here: (1) Dilute the poison in the victim's stomach by having him drink milk or water. (2) Induce vomiting to empty the stomach. (3) Give activated charcoal to absorb the poison that remains in the stomach.

*To induce vomiting.* Have the patient swallow the proper dose of syrup of ipecac: 1 tablespoonful (15 ml.) for a child or 2 tablespoonfuls (30 ml.) for an adult. Follow this by 2 glasses or more of water or milk. If vomiting does not occur within 15 minutes, the first-aider inserts his finger and gently tickles the back of the patient's throat. If syrup of ipecac is not available, have the patient drink fluid and then tickle his throat.

Vomiting should be induced even though it has been several hours since the poison was swallowed. The vomitus should be saved for later examination. If the patient is reclining, turn his head as he vomits so as to prevent choking.

*Activated charcoal* should be administered after the vomiting to absorb what remains of the poison. One or two tablespoonfuls of activated charcoal (powder) are stirred into a glass of water and given to the patient to drink. If the patient vomits again, have him drink another dose of the activated charcoal. Activated charcoal is a harmless potion available at drugstores and is effective in absorbing most poisons and medicines.

# Alphabetical Listing of Specific Poisons

**POISONS**

## BY ACIDS—STRONG ACIDS

Immediately after swallowing a strong acid the victim experiences pain in the mouth, throat, and abdomen. The membranes of the lips and mouth appear white, and the patient experiences intense thirst. If the victim vomits, the vomitus appears as "coffee grounds."

### What to Do

Follow PROCEDURE C on page 334.

## BY ALCOHOL—ETHYL ALCOHOL

(See also *Intoxication, Alcoholic,* page 403, this volume.)

It is this type of alcohol that is contained in alcoholic beverages as well as in many medicines prepared as "tinctures."

Symptoms of poisoning by ethyl alcohol: drunkenness which includes an initial state of excitement, followed by depression, nausea, vomiting, and unconsciousness. When the amount of alcohol in the body fluids becomes dangerously high, the body's vital functions are impaired. When death occurs, it is from paralysis of the breathing mechanism.

### What to Do

1. Cause the patient to vomit as explained under PROCEDURE E on page 334.
2. Keep the patient warm.
3. Make sure that he continues to breathe. Use artificial respiration if necessary. (See *Respiratory Failure,* pages 407-409, this volume.)
4. Give a simple stimulant. If the victim is unconscious, administer strong lukewarm or cold coffee by rectum, in which case the caffeine contained in the coffee will serve as a stimulant.

If the patient is conscious, allow him to drink strong coffee or a glass of water containing one teaspoonful of aromatic spirits of ammonia.

## BY ALCOHOL—METHYL ALCOHOL (Wood Alcohol)

Methyl alcohol is commonly present in paints, paint thinners, paint removers, and "canned heat." One tragic complication of methyl alcohol poisoning is the common occurrence of blindness resulting from damage to the optic nerves.

In addition to the symptoms of intoxication (drunkenness), the victim may have headache, pain in the abdomen, nausea, vomiting, and blindness.

### What to Do

1. Rinse out the victim's stomach by causing him to vomit. See *To Induce Vomiting* under PROCEDURE E, page 334.
2. Protect the patient's eyes from light.
3. Make sure that breathing continues even though this may require artificial respiration. (See *Respiratory Failure,* page 407, this volume.) Administer pure oxygen if available.
4. Arrange for care by a physician or for hospitalization.

## BY ALDRIN *(See By CHLORDANE.)*

## BY AMMONIA

Ammonia is kept commonly about the house to be used as a cleaning agent. When ammonia is swallowed, it causes burning of the mouth, of the esophagus, and of the stomach, followed by thirst and nausea. The fumes of strong ammonia, when blown in the face or when inhaled, cause severe irritation of the membranes of the eyes, throat, and air passages.

### What to Do

Ammonia is a powerful irritant and corrosive. Follow PROCEDURE C on page 334. When the fumes have irritated the eyes, wash the eyes freely

# POISONS

while holding the lids open and using several quarts of water. Afterward the pain may be soothed by placing a few drops of dilute boric acid solution beneath the eyelids.

## BY AMPHETAMINES

The group of amphetamines includes Benzedrine, Dexedrine, and Methedrine. They are used to reduce appetite and weight and to combat fatigue and depression. They are commonly involved in drug abuse under such names as "pep pills," "bennies," and "speed." Overdosage causes serious symptoms and possible death.

### What to Do

Follow PROCEDURE E on page 334.

## BY ANILINE

When aniline has been swallowed, nausea and vomiting occur. Systemic symptoms include shallow breathing, low blood pressure, weak and irregular pulse, convulsions, and unconsciousness.

### What to Do

When aniline has been absorbed through the skin, this skin area should be cleaned with soap and water. If the poison was swallowed, the stomach should be emptied by vomiting. (See *To Induce Vomiting* under PROCEDURE E on page 334.) A dose of Epsom salts (one to two tablespoonfuls in a glass of water) should be given to hasten the removal of the poison from the digestive organs. The victim's most urgent need is an adequate supply of oxygen.

If pure oxygen is available, arrange for the patient to breathe this. If his breathing becomes difficult, use artificial respiration. (See *Respiratory Failure,* page 407, this volume.)

## BY ANTIFREEZE (See By *Ethylene Glycol,* page 339.)

## BY ARSENIC

Arsenic is contained in many insecti-cides, rodent poisons, and crop sprays, as well as in some paints, dyes, and cosmetics.

In the usual case of acute arsenic poisoning the symptoms resemble those of food poisoning. Vomiting may occur within fifteen minutes and intense diarrhea, with watery stools, within one or more hours. There develops a sense of tightness in the throat and of intense pain in the abdomen. There may be muscle cramps, inability to pass urine, unconsciousness, convulsions, and eventual collapse.

### What to Do

Until a trained professional person takes over the case, follow PROCEDURE E on page 334.

The most effective subsequent treatment, to be administered by a physician, is the injection of dimercaprol ("BAL," British antilewisite). This is given by injection in gradually decreasing doses over a period of several days.

## BY ASPIRIN AND OTHER SALICYLATES

Aspirin is the most common cause of poisoning among young children. Symptoms may develop slowly. They include rapid breathing, vomiting, extreme thirst, sweating, fever, and mental confusion. In severe cases there may be unconsciousness or convulsions. Because the symptoms are not distinctive, the diagnosis of aspirin poisoning usually centers around a clue that the child or other victim has taken this drug. When aspirin poisoning is suspected, a physician should be consulted at once.

### What to Do

For the emergency treatment, follow PROCEDURE E on page 334. Call for professional assistance.

## BY ATROPINE, BELLADONNA, AND STRAMONIUM

Atropine eye drops and belladonna preparations occasionlly cause poisoning in children. Stramonium is found in

# First Aid for Emergencies

## What This Chapter Contains

This chapter contains instructions on how to deal with common emergencies until a doctor takes charge of the patient. The material is arranged as indicated in the following skeleton table of contents for the chapter.

In searching for information on any emergency not listed below, please use the General Index at the back of any volume of *You and Your Health*.

Handling an Emergency 349-352
Abdominal Injuries 352, 353
Abrasions 353
Accident, Automobile 353, 354
Artificial Respiration 407-409
Asthma Attack 354, 355
Bandaging Methods 355-361
Bites 362-366
Bleeding 366-368
Breathing Failure 407-409
Bruises 368, 369
Burns 369-373
Cardiac Arrest 373, 374
Cardiopulmonary Resuscitation 374
Chest Injuries 375, 376
Choking 376-379
Cold Injury 379, 380

Coma, Diabetic 418
Convulsions 380
CPR 374, 375
Croup 380
Cuts 380, 381
Delirium 381
Delivery of a Baby 381-384
Dislocations 384-386
Diving, Related Emergencies 386, 387
Drowning 387-389
Electric Shock 410, 411
Emergencies, Handling of 349-352
Epilepsy 380
Fainting 389, 390
Foreign Body Injury 390-392
Fractures 392-396
Frostbite 379, 380
Gunshot Injury 396
Hand Injury 396, 397
Head Injury 397
Heart Attack 397, 398
Heart Stoppage 373, 374
Heat Cramps 399
Heat Exhaustion 399
Heatstroke 399, 400
Hemorrhage 366-368
Hernia, Strangulation of 400, 401
Hiccup 401
Impaction, Fecal 401

E
M
E
R
G
E
N
C
I
E
S

347

Infection 401, 402
Injury, Severe 402
Insanity 402, 403
Intoxication, Alcoholic 403
Lacerations 403, 404
Lightning, Injury by 404
Motion Sickness 404, 405
Mouth-to-Mouth Breathing 407-409
Nosebleed 405
Nuclear Explosion 405, 406
Paralysis 406
Plant Allergies and Poisonings 407
Poisonings 331-346
Rectum, Prolapse of 407
Respiratory Failure 407-409
Shock, Anaphylactic 409
Shock, Circulatory 410
Smoke Inhalation 411, 412
Snakebite 362-365
Spider Bite 365
Spinal Cord Injuries 412
Sports Injuries 412
Sprains 412, 413
Stings 413, 414
Strains 415
Strangling 376-379
Stroke, Apoplectic 415
Suicidal Threat 417
Tarantula Bite 365
Tick Bite 365, 366
Tourniquet 416, 417
Trauma 402
Unconsciousness 417-419
Vomiting 419
Wounds 419
Wounds, Puncture 419, 420

### The Purpose of This Chapter

An emergency is anything that immediately threatens the physical welfare or the life of a person. It is the purpose of this chapter to give concise instruction to persons, not medically trained, on how to render proper emergency care to someone suddenly taken ill or injured.

It is not expected that the reading of this chapter will make anyone proficient enough to take a job in a hospital. Nor will it enable anyone to give all the care that an emergency case may need. In most of the emergency situations considered, however, the suggested care will tide the patient over until a paramedic or a physician can take charge. And this concept typifies the intent of the chapter—to enable any person, medically trained or not, to become a friend in need and thus, perhaps, to save a life.

In many cases of emergency what is not done is just as important to the victim's welfare as what is done. Many times throughout this chapter the reader is warned about what he should *not* do.

The word *emergency* implies to most people that time is of the essence, that what is done must be done at once, that speed at all costs is required. Not necessarily true. A rapid appraisal of the seriousness of a situation is, of course, important. Certain conditions, such as copious bleeding, must be handled quickly and properly before life ebbs away. But in other conditions blind haste may entail greater danger than judicious delay. Many a life has been snuffed out because a person with a broken neck was handled carelessly while being removed from a wrecked car. Often an injured person's prospects of survival are reduced by crowding him into a cramped position in the back seat of a passenger car rather than waiting for an ambulance.

So this chapter is designed to help the person who must handle an emergency to be reasonable in what he does and to act in harmony with the best interests of the victim. Of course you can't carry this big book with you wherever you go. You should, however, prepare yourself for possible emergencies by becoming familiar with the instruction in this chapter, especially if you are interested in first-aid work, if you are active in outdoor recreation, if you or your associates are engaged in hazardous pursuits, or if you are responsible for the welfare of children.

By studying a few items each day and by reviewing a few of the old ones, you will soon become familiar with what to do. This knowledge may enable you to save life—possibly at some unexpected time, possibly soon.

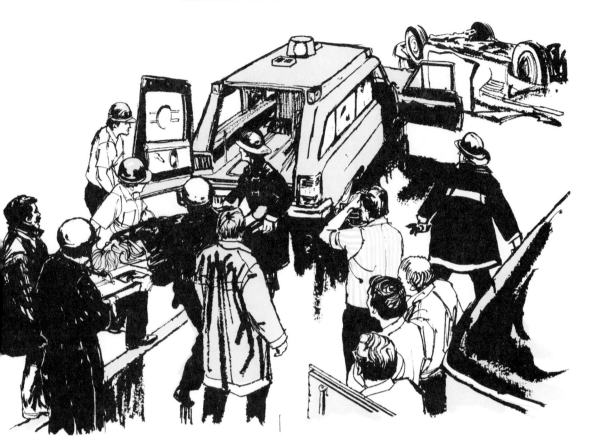

**Possibility of an unexpected automobile accident challenges every
citizen to preparedness as a first-aider.**

### First Things to Do in a
### Grave Emergency

Persons suddenly injured or stricken with illness do not have labels on them telling what the trouble is and what help should be given. So the person who renders aid must evaluate the circumstances and the condition of the victim and decide what to do. The better trained this person is and the more careful and accurate his observations, the better care he will be able to give. Suppose that *you* are the person who must give emergency care to someone suddenly taken sick or injured. Don't waste time in bemoaning your lack of training. Get on with the job and do the best you can; that is all that can be expected of anyone.

If other people are around, you may ask yourself, Am I the best qualified to give aid? If not, then let the better qualified person take charge while you follow his instructions. But unless you know that someone else can render better emergency care than you can, take over and tell others what to do without thought of hurt feelings. If someone else tries to replace you, question his qualifications. You be the judge of who is best able to give emergency care. While in charge, do not let others disregard your instructions. Use a firm voice, and ask for the help you need.

The following suggestions are intended to help you think logically when handling an emergency.

A. *Keep calm.* Even though you feel

349

nervous, put on the act of being calm and deliberate. This will help you to think clearly and will help the victim, if conscious, to avoid psychological panic that might throw him into shock. Keeping calm also inspires the confidence of those helping you.

B. *If the emergency consists of a sudden illness,* try to get in touch with a doctor. Send someone else to phone while you continue caring for the victim. Have this person tell the doctor about the circumstances and the victim's present condition and ask for advice on what to do. If a doctor cannot be reached, direct the call to the emergency room of a hospital.

C. *When poison has been swallowed,* place an emergency call at once for a physician, the emergency squad of the fire department, or a poison control center. Preferably this call should be placed by a second responsible person so that the first-aider can devote all his time to the care of the patient. In placing the call, give as much information as possible: the patient's name, any clue as to the nature of the poison (such as the wording on the label on the container), the patient's symptoms, and the patient's exact location. The person placing the call should ask for instructions on how to care for the patient until help arrives or while the patient is being taken to an emergency room. For further information on first aid for poisoning, see the previous chapter, beginning on page 333.

D. *When the victim has been burned,* follow the instructions beginning on page 369 of this chapter, on how to care for the particular kind of burn with which you are concerned.

E. *In case of an accident,* it may be more important to have someone call an ambulance than to phone for a doctor. Ambulance crews are trained in first aid and therefore can do the best for the victim while taking him to the nearest hospital. If you are in an isolated area where an ambulance cannot reach you soon, call for a policeman or a sheriff.

F. *Don't be in a hurry to move an injured person* unless it is essential for his safety. First, try to determine the nature of the problem. In some serious illnesses and injuries, moving the victim without proper equipment or before first aid is rendered may cause death. Do not allow the injured person to sit up, much less to stand or try to walk.

G. *When a person is not breathing,* begin giving artificial respiration at once. This is of first priority, for one may die within a matter of three or four minutes without air. Mouth-to-mouth breathing, in which you force your own breath into the patient's mouth and thus into his lungs (while holding his nostrils closed), is the simplest and most effective method of artificial respiration. For further instruction on giving artificial respiration, see the item RESPIRATORY FAILURE beginning on page 407 of this chapter.

H. *Next in importance is to check for bleeding.* The simplest way to control continued loss of large amounts of blood from an injured part is to place a clean cloth right into the wound and exert firm, continuous pressure. For additional instruction on the control of bleeding, see the item BLEEDING beginning on page 366 of this chapter.

I. *When the victim is unconscious,* care for him as best you can right where you are until conditions are favorable for moving him. Make sure that he continues to breathe, either naturally or by artificial respiration. Don't try to rouse an unconscious person. Don't try to give him fluids by mouth. Remove loose objects such as false teeth so that these will not interfere with his breathing. Keep him covered to conserve his body heat. For further information see the item UNCONSCIOUSNESS in this chapter beginning on page 417.

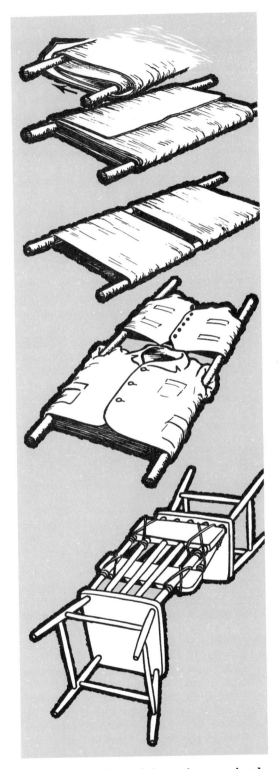

J. *Look for evidences of fractured bones.* The most serious possibility here is that of a broken neck or a broken back. See the item FRAC-TURES beginning on page 392 of this chapter.

K. *General care of the waiting victim.* While waiting for instructions from a doctor or while waiting for the ambulance to arrive, follow certain principles of general care such as these:

1. Loosen tight clothing which may constrict the victim's neck or waist.

2. Do not administer any form of alcoholic drink.

3. Conserve body heat by covering the victim with a blanket or with coats. Be mindful of the danger of burning the skin of an unconscious person by the use of heating devices. (See the item SHOCK beginning on page 410 of this chapter, and the item CIRCULATORY SHOCK in chapter 9, volume 2.)

4. When the victim vomits, turn his head gently to one side to avoid the danger of his choking on the vomitus. If he is lying on the ground, dig a little trench into which the vomitus may flow or lay a sheet of newspaper beside his head. Using a handkerchief or paper tissue, gently wipe away the remaining vomitus from the victim's face and lips.

L. *When the time comes to move the victim,* take care so as not to change the relative position of the parts of his body. His body should be kept straight and horizontal, not allowed to sag, jackknife, or twist. If the victim must be moved from where his body rests on the highway, he can be slid lengthwise on a blanket. The blanket for this sledding purpose can be placed under the victim by rolling him gently to one side while half of the blanket is tucked under him. Then, by rolling him to the opposite side, the tucked portion of the blanket may be straightened.

Another way of transporting an injured or very sick person is by the use of an improvised stretcher made from two poles placed through the arms of two jackets, the jacket arms having

**Examples of how improvised stretchers for moving an accident victim can be made.**

351

EMERGENCIES

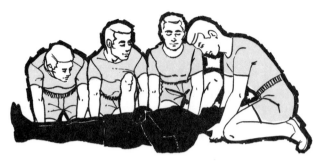

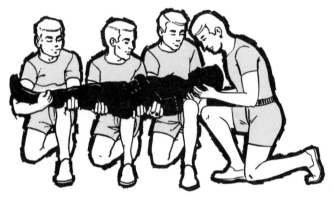

Cooperative effort, carefully synchronized, is essential in moving the victim of an accident.

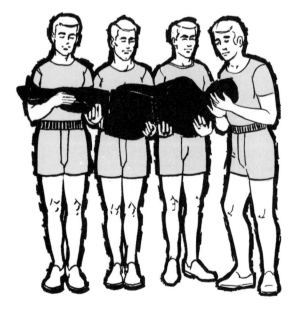

been turned wrong side out.

Still another proper way to move an injured person is by the cooperative effort of four persons who work carefully together as they lift and move the victim. Three take their position on one side of the victim, one at his shoulder, one at his hip, and one at his knees. If one side is injured, they work from the uninjured side. The fourth person is located at the victim's head, and his one responsibility is to lift the head in unison with the other three persons in such a way that the head does not change position in relation to the victim's shoulders.

# Common Emergencies and Emergency Procedures

## ABDOMINAL INJURIES

We consider here injuries sustained by violence in which the abdominal wall has been torn open or has sustained a stab wound. Gunshot wounds are considered on page 396 of this same chapter.

Abdominal injuries are serious because of the possibility of damage to the abdominal organs, the possibility of hemorrhage within the abdominal cavity, and the grave danger of infection of the organs and tissues within the abdomen. Every abdominal injury requires careful examination by a physician and definitive treatment which often involves surgical exploration. The function of the first-aider is to care for the victim until an ambulance arrives or the patient is received at a hospital emergency room.

### What to Do

**1. Keep the victim lying flat on his back with a pad under his knees so as to relax the muscles of the abdominal wall.**

**2. If the intestines protrude through the abdominal wound, the first-aider should not try to return these to their normal position but should protect the exposed tissue by covering with a clean cloth, a piece of clean plastic, or a sheet of metal foil.**

tack than with the long-range cure of the disease. For additional information, consult the General Index for the item, *Asthma*.

If the patient has had previous asthmatic attacks, he probably has learned to use a medication for the control of his symptoms. If so, this medication should now be administered to relieve the acute attack.

For the immediate treatment of asthma, other than by medication, try giving the patient a drink of hot milk, Postum, or just plain hot water. This may relax the tissues in the air passages.

A steam inhalation accompanied by a hot foot bath may bring relief. If no mechanical vaporizer is available, moist air may be provided by conducting steam from a pan of boiling water through a paper cone to the area of the patient's face. Care must be taken not to burn the face or the sensitive membranes of the nose.

If these simple remedies do not relieve the attack, a physician should be consulted by phone, or the patient should be taken to a hospital emergency room where he can receive such medication as epinephrine which will relieve the obstruction in the air passages.

## BANDAGING METHODS

*Why a Bandage?* A bandage is an external cover designed to protect an injury from contamination during the healing process. Examples are the small, ready-prepared adhesive bandage available at the drugstore; or its larger counterpart, a sterile gauze bandage designed to be held in place by a cloth wrapping. A bandage may also be used in cases of fracture or deep injury to hold splints in place or to prevent movement of the injured part. Another use is to exert firm pressure on the underlying tissues, helpful, for example, in the control of bleeding.

*Principles of Bandaging.* A bandage should be snug but not so tight as to impede the circulation of blood. Even for one experienced in bandaging, the question of how tight is so difficult to answer that he may have to remove and replace a bandage a time or two in order to find the happy medium. Even then, the swelling of tissues may decline and the bandage become too loose, or the injured tissues may swell and the bandage become too tight. A bandage applied to the leg, the arm, or the finger should be double-checked occasionally to make sure the tissues beyond the bandage are warm and of normal color.

When a bandage is used to hold a wet dressing in place, the cloth of which the bandage is made may become moist and shrink and thus make the bandage tighter. This possibility emphasizes again the need for occasional checking.

It may be advisable to place strips of adhesive tape over a bandage to keep it from shifting. These can extend beyond the bandage so as to anchor it to the skin. The loose end of the bandage can be fastened either by the use of adhesive tape or, in the case of a roller bandage, by tearing or cutting the bandage down the center for a few inches, tying the loose ends together with a simple knot, and then using them as straps, one passing in one direction and one the other, to serve as a final tie.

*Kinds of Bandages:*

A. *The Roller Bandage.* This is made of muslin cloth or of gauze prepared especially for bandages and designed to stretch slightly so that it conforms to the shape of the part being bandaged. Roller bandage material, because usually sterile when packaged, can be applied safely to a wound which has been cleansed. Roller bandage material comes in various widths from about one-half inch to four inches, the narrower widths being used for fingers and toes. The accompanying drawings indicate how roller bandages can be applied to various parts of the body.

Roller bandages may need to be reinforced by the use of adhesive strips, either to hold the roller bandage in place or to add support to the injured part as,

355

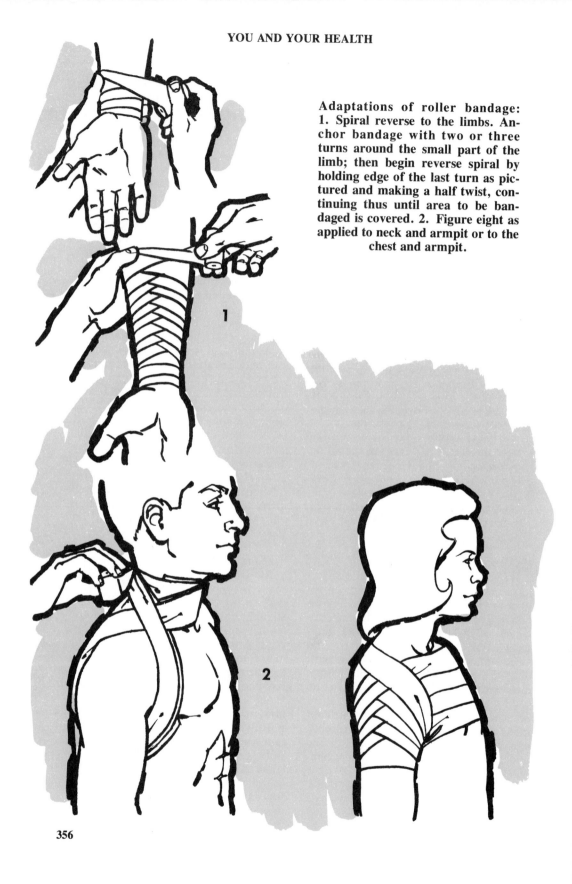

Adaptations of roller bandage: 1. Spiral reverse to the limbs. Anchor bandage with two or three turns around the small part of the limb; then begin reverse spiral by holding edge of the last turn as pictured and making a half twist, continuing thus until area to be bandaged is covered. 2. Figure eight as applied to neck and armpit or to the chest and armpit.

Roller bandages continued: 3. Figure eight to the elbow. This is especially suitable whenever a single bandage needs to be applied above, across, and below the elbow or knee. 4. Multiple cranial.

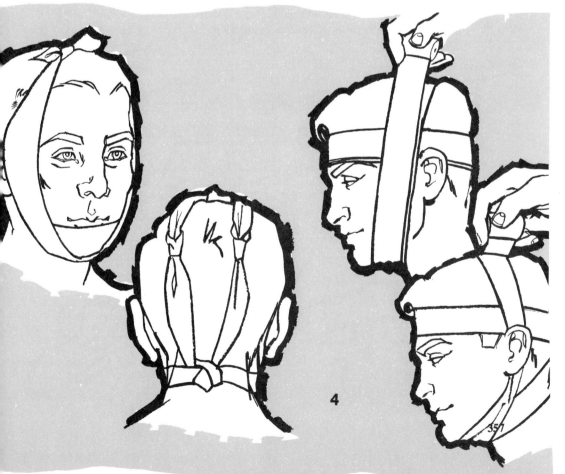

3

4

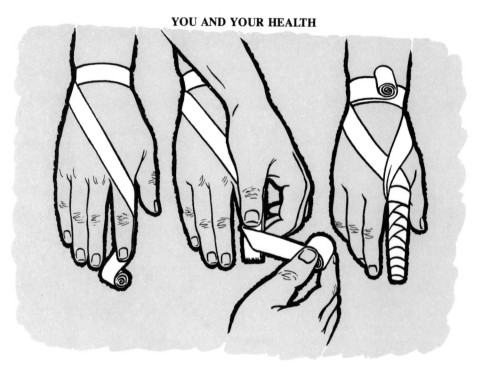

Narrow widths of roller bandages
can be used effectively for bandaging a finger, the spiral and recurrent loop technique being used.

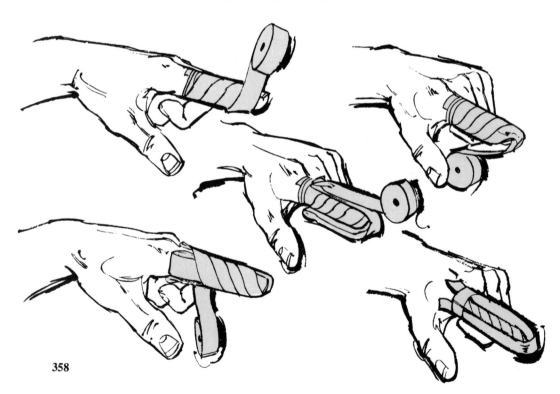

358

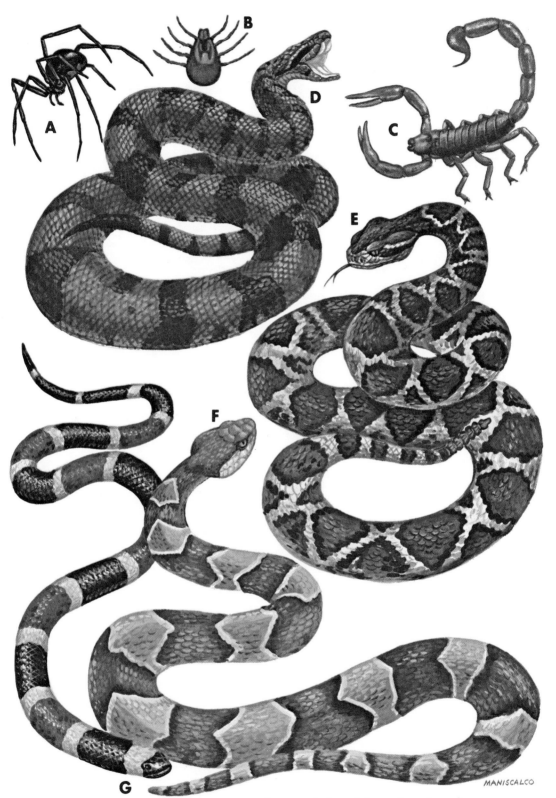

A. Black widow spider (note characteristic red hourglass-shaped mark on underside of the abdomen); B. tick; C. scorpion; D. cottonmouth; E. rattlesnake; F. copperhead; and G. coral snake.

363

EMERGENCIES

# FIRST AID FOR SNAKEBITE

## POISONOUS OR NONPOISONOUS

Poisonous or nonpoisonous, a snakebite should have medical attention. A snakebite victim should be taken to a hospital *as quickly as possible*, even in cases when snakebite is only suspected.

## FIRST AID

1. As stated above, *get the victim to a hospital fast.* Meanwhile, take the following general first aid measures:
   - Keep the victim from moving around.
   - Keep the victim as calm as possible, preferably lying down.
   - Immobilize the bitten extremity and keep it at or below heart level.

   If a hospital can be reached within 4 to 5 hours and no symptoms develop, this is all that is necessary.

2. *If mild to moderate symptoms develop, apply a constricting band* from 2 to 4 inches above the bite but NOT around a joint (i.e., elbow, knee, wrist, or ankle) and NOT around the head, neck, or trunk. The band should be from ¾ to 1½ inches wide, NOT thin like a rubber band. The band should be snug, but loose enough to slip one finger underneath. Be alert to swelling; loosen the band if it becomes too tight, but do not remove it. To ensure that blood flow has not been stopped, periodically check the pulse in the extremity beyond the bite.

3. *If severe symptoms develop, incisions and suction should be performed immediately.* Apply a constricting band, if not already done, and make a cut in the skin with a sharp sterilized blade through the fang mark(s). Cuts should be no deeper than just through the skin and should be ½ inch long, extending over the suspected venom deposit point (because a snake strikes downward, the deposit point is usually lower than the fang mark). Cuts should be made along the long axis of the limb. DO NOT make cross-cut incisions; DO NOT make cuts on the head, neck, or trunk. Suction should be applied with a suction cup for 30 minutes. If a suction cup is not available, use the mouth. There is little risk to the rescuer who uses his mouth, but it is recommended that the venom not be swallowed and that the mouth be rinsed.

## IF THE HOSPITAL IS NOT CLOSE (cannot be reached within from 4 to 5 hours)

1. Continue to try to obtain professional care by transportation of the victim or by communication with a rescue service.
2. *If no symptoms develop,* continue trying to reach the hospital and give the general first aid described above.
3. *If ANY symptoms develop,* apply a constricting band and perform incisions and suction immediately, as described above.

## OTHER CONSIDERATIONS

1. *Shock:* Keep the victim lying down and comfortable and maintain body temperature.
2. *Breathing and heartbeat:* If breathing stops, give mouth-to-mouth resuscitation. If breathing stops and there is no pulse, cardiopulmonary resuscitation (CPR) should be performed by those trained to do so.
3. *Identifying the snake:* If the snake can be killed without risk or delay, it should be brought, *with care,* to the hospital for identification.
4. *Cleansing the bitten area:* The bitten area may be washed with soap and water and blotted dry with sterile gauze. Dressings and bandages can be applied, but only for a short period of time.
5. *Cold therapy:* Cold compresses, ice, dry ice, chemical ice packs, spray refrigerants, and other methods of cold therapy are NOT recommended in the first aid treatment of snakebite.
6. *Medicine to relieve pain:* A medicine *not containing aspirin* can be given to the victim for relief of pain. DO NOT give alcohol, sedatives, aspirin, or other medications.
7. *Snakebite kits:* Keep a kit accessible for all outings in snake-infested or primitive areas.

## SYMPTOMS

1. *Mild to moderate* symptoms include mild swelling or discoloration and mild to moderate pain at the wound site with tingling sensations, rapid pulse, weakness, dimness of vision, nausea, vomiting, and shortness of breath.
2. *Severe* symptoms include rapid swelling and numbness, followed by severe pain at the wound site. Other effects include pinpoint pupils, twitching, slurred speech, shock, convulsions, paralysis, unconsciousness, and no breathing or pulse.

The information on this poster is based on a report prepared for the American Red Cross by the National Academy of Sciences-National Research Council.

## American Red Cross

Snakebite prevention practices that can eliminate needless illness and worry may be learned in a Red Cross first aid course. Call your chapter to enroll.

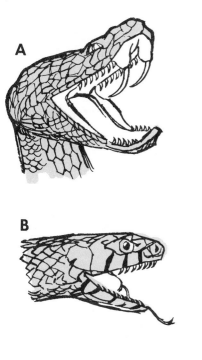

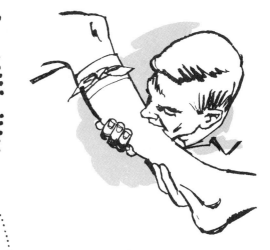

Emergency treatment for snakebite includes suction of wound. This can be done by mouth after making an X-shaped incision across the fang marks left by the bite.

Bite of pit viper (A) compared with bite of a nonpoisonous snake (B). Note two characteristic fang marks in former, plus tooth marks; but in latter no fang marks, only six rows of tooth marks.

C. *Spider Bite.* The spider which causes the greatest discomfort and harm is the female black widow spider, found throughout the Americas. The bite produces a sharp pain locally, followed in about thirty minutes by rigidity of the muscles of the abdomen and abdominal cramps. Weakness, severe pain in the limbs, and even convulsions (especially in children) may come later. The outcome depends on the amount of venom injected, the general vitality of the victim, and the promptness with which treatment is administered. The mortality rate is about 5 percent, with most deaths occurring in children.

### What to Do

1. Take the victim to a hospital as quickly as possible. Local treatment at the site of the spider bite is not effective.

2. Warm baths may help to relieve the muscle pain.

3. Antivenin prepared especially for black widow spider bites should be injected intramuscularly as promptly as possible.

D. *Tarantula Bite.* Tarantula bites may be painful but are usually less serious than bites by the black widow spider.

### What to Do

1. For a minor involvement, apply cold compresses to the area of the bite.

2. For a more serious involvement in which systemic symptoms develop, apply a constricting band to the affected arm or leg as described in item 2 of First Aid for Snakebite on page 364. Be prepared to give artificial respiration by the mouth-to-mouth method if necessary to keep the victim breathing (see pages 407-409).

E. *Tick Bites.* The bite of a tick not only produces discomfort in the local area where the tick's head is buried in the skin, but it may also transmit infections, some of which are serious.

### What to Do

In attempting to remove a tick, one risks the danger that the body will break away, leaving the head still embedded in the skin. To avoid this, turpentine may be applied to the exposed portion of the tick. Or, touching the tick with an extinguished matchhead (still hot) may cause the insect to release its grasp. Another method is to cover the tick and the skin immediately surrounding it with petrolatum (vaseline) or heavy oil. This closes the insect's breathing pores, usually forcing it to dislodge within half an hour. As a last resort, the insect may be removed from the skin by careful manipulation with tweezers, rotating the head counterclockwise.

Following removal, the skin area should be scrubbed with soap and water for about five minutes. If the victim develops a fever within the next few hours, a physician should be consulted, because this symptom may indicate that the tick has transmitted disease-producing germs.

### BLEEDING (HEMORRHAGE)

The control of severe bleeding is important as a life-saving measure.

There are two main kinds of bleeding: external and internal. In external bleeding, blood escapes to the outside as when tissues are torn by a cut or by crushing injury. In internal bleeding, blood escapes from a blood vessel into the tissues or into one of the body cavities. A person may die from internal bleeding even though not a drop of blood escapes to the outside.

A person may lose as much as two or three pints of blood and still survive. If a large artery has been severed and bleeding is rapid, it does not take long for this much blood to be lost. The treatment of such bleeding, therefore, must be prompt.

The loss of significant amounts of blood, whether it be by external bleed-ing or internal bleeding, causes certain changes in the body functions. These occur even in a case of internal bleeding and may serve as an aid in determining that bleeding is taking place. For these general symptoms of bleeding, see chapter 6, volume 2. For the meaning of bleeding as it occurs in various parts of the body, see the General Index and the subheadings under the entry *Bleeding.*

A. *External Bleeding.* An injured person should be examined completely as soon as possible to determine whether he is losing blood. Clothing must be removed from parts of the body where blood is seen seeping through.

### What to Do

1. Apply direct pressure at the point of bleeding. A sterile gauze dressing, a clean sanitary napkin, or a freshly laundered piece of cloth should be placed over or into the wound and held there firmly. Only the amount of pressure necessary to stop the bleeding should be used, for excessive pressure may interfere with the blood supply to other parts. If such pressure controls the bleeding, a bandage may be necessary to hold the temporary dressing in place until the patient reaches the hospital. When pressure over the wound does not control the bleeding, see the next item.

2. Use pressure points to control persistent bleeding, particularly when blood comes in spurts as when an artery has been severed. The accompanying diagram shows the locations in the body where the arteries run near enough to the surface to be closed off by pressure from the outside. Bleeding from a large artery will seldom stop of its own accord, for the flow of blood is too brisk to permit the formation of a blood clot. In such a case, pressure over the proper pressure point may need to be maintained until a physician ties off the bleeding artery. Obviously, the control of bleeding at a pressure point applies only to

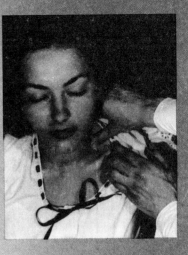

Position of the five pressure points of the body, at which persistent bleeding from an artery may be controlled if direct pressure at wound fails to stop bleeding. This method may be used only to control bleeding from the arms, legs, or face, not from other parts of the body.

bleeding from an arm, a leg, or the face. Do not try to control the bleeding of the head, neck, or body by applying pressure at pressure points.

3. Apply a tourniquet as a LAST RESORT when severe bleeding from an arm or a leg cannot be controlled by the methods mentioned above. Use of a tourniquet can result in permanent injury to the arm or leg, with the probability of amputation. If blood is being lost so rapidly, however, as to endanger life, it is better to run the risk of amputation than to permit the victim to bleed to death. A wide band of cloth such as is used for a bandage or such as may be torn from a sheet or a shirt is folded to make a strip three or four inches wide and consisting of about four layers of cloth. This is wrapped snugly twice around the bleeding arm or leg. It should be placed as close as possible to the bleeding wound, between it and the victim's heart. The free ends of the band of cloth should be tied with an overhand knot. A short, strong stick or similar article that will not break is placed on the knot and two additional overhand knots are tied on top of the stick so as to hold it in place. The stick is then twisted, tightening the tourniquet, until bleeding stops. One or both ends of the stick are then tied to the limb in such a way that the twisting cannot unwind.

See the item TOURNIQUET in this same chapter, pages 416, 417.

When a tourniquet is applied to an injured person, written notation should accompany the patient to the hospital indicating that a tourniquet has been applied and the time of application. The information can be written on the victim's forehead with an indelible pencil or lipstick if no paper is available. The tourniquet should remain exposed where it may be seen by hospital attendants and not forgotten.

4. Prevent or treat shock. Excessive loss of blood increases the probability of shock. As a precaution, the patient should be placed in a reclining position and kept comfortably warm. If bleeding is from an arm or a leg, this part should be elevated so as to reduce the blood pressure in it and thus favor control of the bleeding. If the victim is conscious, encourage him to take liquids by mouth. Avoid coffee, however, or any other stimulant, because stimulants raise the blood pressure and thus increase the tendency to bleed.

B. *Internal Hemorrhage.* Internal hemorrhage results from damage to or rupture of one of the internal organs such as the liver or spleen; from the rupture of an oviduct (as in tubal pregnancy); from the severing of a blood vessel (as in gunshot); from disease within a lung; from rupture of varicose veins in the esophagus; or from erosion into a blood vessel as by an ulcer in the stomach or intestine.

Bleeding from the lungs is usually indicated by coughing up of bright-red, frothy blood. Bleeding from the stomach may be indicated by vomited blood—red if the blood is recent, and dark and clotted if the blood has been acted on by the digestive juices. Bleeding into the intestine may be evidenced by the passing of jet-black stools. Bleeding near the anal opening causes the stools to be streaked with bright-red blood.

### What to Do

Often the only adequate treatment for severe internal bleeding is appropriate surgery. While waiting for the doctor, the victim should be kept warm, with his feet and legs elevated above the level of his body to prevent or control the condition of shock.

## BRUISES (CONTUSIONS)

A bruise, or contusion, is an injury to the deeper tissues in which the skin is usually not broken. It could be caused by a blow from a fist or a club, by a pinch, or by impact against a solid object as in falling or in being struck by some moving object. In a typical case the small blood vessels are broken in

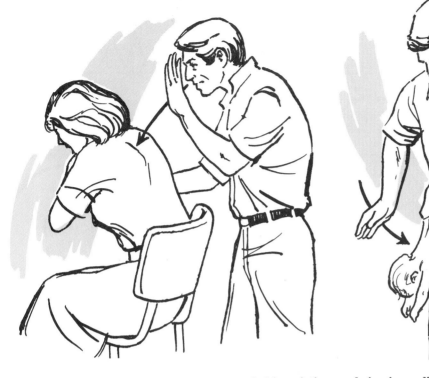

Delivering back blows to a choking victim can bring immediate relief if the obstruction is not lodged too firmly. Notice the method for handling an infant.

maneuvers: (1) *Back Blows*, (2) *Epigastric Thrust* (the Heimlich maneuver), and (3) *Finger Probe*. Any one of these may work successfully in a given case.

1. *Back Blows*. This maneuver requires the operator to use the heel of his hand to deliver a series of rapid whacks to the victim's spine between his shoulder blades. The maneuver may be used with the victim standing, sitting, or lying on his side. The blow should be forceful enough to jar the victim's body and thus dislodge the object obstructing his air passages. A gentle modification of the maneuver may be used in the case of an infant by supporting the infant, face down, on one's forearm (see accompanying illustration). Only when he is unable to breathe at all should his head be held low.

2. *Epigastric Thrust (the Heimlich maneuver)*. Some air remains within the lungs even when a person's air passages are closed as in choking. The epigastric thrust maneuver is designed to force this residual air out of the lungs so quickly that it pushes the material trapped in the throat upward into the mouth, thus removing the hindrance to the flow of air. This maneuver is accomplished by exerting swift pressure upward through the soft tissue of the epigastrium. The epigastrium is that part of the front portion of the body wall located just below the breastbone and between the lower ribs as they curve downward and outward. Such pressure forces the diaphragm upward, thus compressing the lungs and forcing the air upward through the air passages.

The maneuver can be performed with the victim standing, sitting, or

377

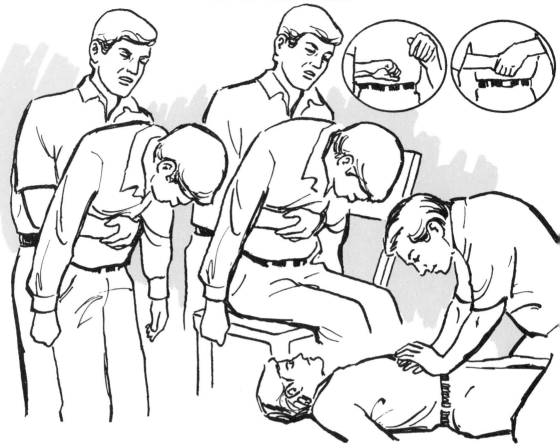

lying on his back. When the choking person is standing or sitting, the operator works from behind. He wraps his arm around the victim's waist, placing the thumb side of one fist against the victim's abdomen just above the navel and just below the ribs. He then grabs his fist with his other hand and makes a quick upward thrust (see accompanying illustrations).

When the victim is lying on his back, the epigastric thrust is performed as the operator kneels beside the victim or straddles the victim's hips. He places one of his hands on top of the other with the heel of the lower hand located slightly above the victim's navel and just below the ribs. The operator then rocks forward as he makes a quick upward thrust in the midline of the victim's body.

3. *Finger Probe*. This maneuver is especially useful when it is certain that a bolus of food or other firm object has become lodged in the victim's throat. Open the victim's mouth widely, grasp the tip of his tongue through the fold of a handkerchief, and pull the tongue well forward. Pass the forefinger of the other hand over the tongue and along the side (not the middle) of the victim's throat far enough to reach the edge of the obstructing object. (If the finger were pushed into the midline of the victim's throat, it migh push the obstructing object farther into the air passages.) Then with a sweeping motion, bring the object forward into the victim's mouth.

After the choking victim has received first aid, even though he appears to be breathing normally again,

The epigastric thrust (opposite page) or the finger probe (above) may be required to dislodge obstructions which cannot be removed by blows to the back. In using the finger probe, care must be taken to prevent pushing the obstruction farther into the air passages.

it is important that he be seen by a physician. The reason for this imperative is to determine whether the obstruction to the airways has been completely removed and whether the maneuvers used to restore his breathing have caused any damage to his tissues.

### COLD INJURY (FROSTBITE)

Cold injury so severe as to cause freezing of the tissues is called frostbite. It may occur in such exposed parts of the body as the ears, nose, hands, or feet. Just before the tissues become frozen, they may appear violet-red in color. Once freezing has occurred, color changes to gray-yellow.

#### What to Do

1. Avoid rubbing the frozen parts, and do not resort to the outmoded treatment of massaging with snow to bring about thawing.

2. After placing the victim in a warm room, remove all items of clothing that constrict the frozen part of the body, such as boots, gloves, or socks.

3. Immerse the frozen part in warm water (not hot) and attempt to raise the temperature of the frozen tissues gradually to normal body temperature. When the nose or the ear is frozen, use compresses wrung from warm water to thaw the frozen part.

4. Try to improve the victim's general condition by keeping him warm and giving him hot drinks (not liquor).

5. After the frozen part has thawed, keep it dry and avoid the use of wet dressings.

6. Take special precautions to

379

avoid pressure of heavy bedclothing or other objects against the part that was frozen. The part may need to be protected by a "cradle" placed over it, keeping the bedclothes from touching it.

7. Encourage the victim to move the part that was frozen, for this will increase blood circulation through these tissues. If it was his foot, he should avoid standing on it until the tissues are completely healed.

## CONVULSIONS (EPILEPSY)

A consideration of the convulsive disorders, their significance and causes, appears in chapter 4, volume 3. In the present chapter we are concerned with the first-aid handling of a person who has a convulsion.

### What to Do

1. Place the victim on something wide and soft such as a bed or a thick rug so that he will not be injured on account of his involuntary motions—if on a bed, stand guard so that he will not fall off.

2. Loosen his clothing so as to reduce the danger of choking or harm caused by the twisting of garments.

3. Put something blunt and soft (such as a small roll of cloth) between the victim's teeth so as to hold the jaws apart and thus reduce the danger of his biting his tongue.

4. Place the victim on his side rather than on his back, for, particularly in the case of a child, danger of vomiting exists and the possibility that he may choke on the vomitus. Do not leave the patient face down because of the danger of smothering. Always keep his face turned to one side.

5. Breathing is usually interrupted for brief periods during a convulsion. If breathing stops completely for more than a minute or two, administer artificial respiration. See the item RESPIRATORY FAILURE on pages 407-409 of this same chapter.

NOTE: Do *not* put anyone with convulsions in the bathtub. The

thrashing movements of the convulsion can cause injuries here. Furthermore, it is difficult to care for a person in a bathtub.

6. In convulsions associated with high fever, as in cases of heatstroke or the beginning of an illness marked by fever, take measures to reduce the body temperature as quickly as possible. This is best done by wrapping the patient in a sheet wrung out of cold water. Then allow an electric fan to play on the wet sheet. This will cause rapid evaporation of the moisture in the sheet and will have a cooling effect. Cool sponging of the victim's skin with a damp cloth produces a similar effect.

7. Convulsions not associated with fever typically last for only a short time. The first-aider's effort in such a case is to protect the victim so that he will not injure himself during the convulsion. After the convulsion the individual should be permitted to rest quietly until he feels reasonably normal again.

8. When repeated convulsions occur, one after the other, arrange for medical help or transport the patient to the emergency room of a hospital.

## CROUP

See chapter 17, volume 1, for a discussion on croup.

## CUTS

A cut, in contrast to a puncture wound, usually lies open, bleeds easily, and is less likely to become infected. Such a wound is caused by a knife, a razor, broken glass, or any sharp edge.

### What to Do

Treatment depends on the size and location of the cut. Simple cuts can be safely treated at home. Deeper or more extensive cuts, particularly those in which nerves and blood vessels may be involved, require the services of a physician. For simple cuts, care may be given as follows:

1. Bleeding should be controlled first. In simple cases, firm pressure

disturbances of vision, and dizziness—these beginning to appear soon after the diver emerges from the water.

### What to Do

**Treatment of decompression sickness involves use of pressure equipment, which may not be easily available. Official lifeguards and other authorities in areas where diving is common are usually informed on the location of such equipment and can help in transporting the victim to such a center.**

**In treating decompression sickness, the victim is placed in a tank constructed for this purpose and the air pressure within the tank is increased to simulate the pressure to which he was subjected while diving. The pressure is then gradually reduced, over a period of a few hours, allowing the patient's tissues to make a gradual adjustment.**

## DROWNING

Drowning is listed as America's fourth leading cause of accidental death, accounting for about 7000 casualties per year.

A swimmer in danger of drowning often panics. He thus makes it dangerous for another swimmer, even though skilled, to rescue him lest he cling to his rescuer so tenaciously as to pull him under too. It is better therefore to throw an imperiled swimmer a rope or a life preserver than to attempt a person-to-person rescue, or perhaps reach for him with an oar or pole.

If the person in danger has been injured while in the water, great caution should be used in removing him. It is relatively easy to keep the average person afloat with his mouth and nose above water; however, once attempt is made to remove him, the buoyancy which the water imparts is lost and the struggle to lift him may even aggravate his injury. It is best to keep an injured person afloat until suitable equipment arrives, even though this may mean administering mouth-to-mouth respiration while the victim is still in the water. The acceptable way to remove an injured person from the water is to place a firm stretcher or wooden door or wide plank underneath him to keep his body straight while he is being lifted out of the water.

Many factors may contribute to the hazard of drowning, even with experienced swimmers. One, formerly mysterious but now understood, is hyperventilation. This danger threatens a swimmer when he takes several deep breaths just before swimming underwater, thereby releasing from his body a large portion of carbon dioxide which, under normal circumstances, would stimulate his continued breathing. Thus the swimmer loses his desire to breathe and falls in danger of losing consciousness while still holding his breath. Another circumstance in which this same tragic series of events may occur is that of diving repeatedly with very short intervals between dives. Here again the diver may breathe so vigorously between dives as to nearly rid his body of carbon dioxide and thus lose his urge to breathe to the extent that he loses consciousness while under water and fails to surface for another breath.

### What to Do

**If there is anyone else at the scene, send him at once to summon help, preferably a rescue squad. Do not leave the victim yourself, but stay with him and keep him breathing.**

**1. Keep the victim breathing. This is the rescuer's primary occupation, and he must work to this end even while the victim is still in the water and even later while he is being taken to the hospital. If the victim is still breathing on his own, well and good. If not, artificial respiration must be administered as outlined below.**

**2. Begin artificial respiration at once if the victim is not breathing. Allow not more than 10 seconds for clearing debris or mucus or water out of the victim's mouth and then begin mouth-to-mouth resuscitation.**

**3. Place the victim's head in exten-**

387

EMERGENCIES

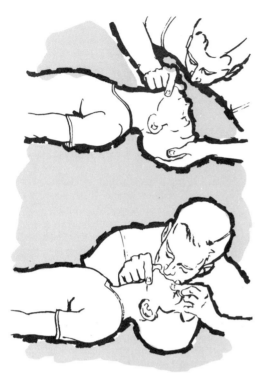

In mouth-to-mouth artificial respiration the victim's chin is kept tilted upward. (For other illustrations of this method see *Respiratory Failure* in this chapter.)

sion (chin up) as illustrated in the accompanying drawing. This tends to keep the air passages open so that air can enter his lungs.

4. Fill your own lungs with air and then breathe this into the victim's mouth while holding his nostrils closed either by your cheek against the openings or by your thumb and finger. This forced air should cause the victim's chest to expand. If the victim is a child, remember that the capacity of his lungs is small. Be careful, therefore, not to overinflate them, but give small, short puffs. Do not waste time trying to get water out of the victim's lungs before you begin to breathe into his mouth.

5. If the victim's mouth is clenched shut, as sometimes occurs in the case of a drowning person, separate his lips and breathe into his mouth anyway, allowing your breath to pass between his teeth. After filling the victim's lungs with your own breath, take your mouth away while he expels this air. This he will do on his own without your having to compress his chest and even though he is unconscious.

6. Be alert to the possibility that the victim may vomit. If he does, simply turn his head to one side, clean out his mouth as quickly as possible, and continue breathing air into his lungs. Vomiting simply indicates that the victim is short on oxygen. Furthermore, he may have swallowed considerable water, which is now being regurgitated.

7. It is common for a drowning person to have a convulsion. Do not let this alarm you, and do not let it interrupt the mouth-to-mouth resuscitation any longer than absolutely necessary.

8. When the rescue squad arrives, allow those with experience to take over giving artificial respiration, a task sometimes accomplished by a mechanical device administering pure oxygen to the victim.

9. While continuing mouth-to-mouth respiration, feel high on the side of the victim's neck for the pulsation of his carotid arteries. If you feel none, presumably the victim's heart has stopped. It then becomes necessary for you or someone helping you to stimulate heart action. This is done by applying pressure over the lower third of the victim's breastbone, releasing it, and exerting it again in a rhythm of about one cycle per second. The amount of pressure to be applied varies with the age of the victim. For babies, the pressure should be gentle, exerted through the tips of the operator's fingers as they press against the center of the baby's breastbone. For children of about 10 years of age, pressure should be exerted by the heel of one hand. For adults, one of the operator's hands is placed over the other so that pressure is exerted by

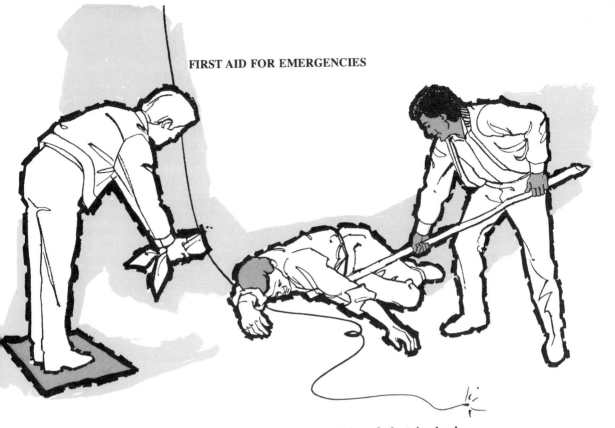

Precaution to be observed in removing a victim of electric shock from contact with the current: Rescuer should insulate himself by use of a dry wooden pole, rubber sheet, or dry cloth and prevent grounding by standing on a dry board.

start mouth-to-mouth type of artificial respiration at once and continue as long as he does not breathe spontaneously (even while en route to the hospital) or until a physician pronounces him dead. (See the item RESPIRATORY FAILURE on pages 407-409 of this same chapter.)

4. If the victim's heart is not beating, see the items CARDIAC ARREST and CARDIOPULMONARY RESUSCITATION on pages 373 and 374 of this same chapter.

5. Even after the victim has resumed breathing, keep him quiet, warm, and lying down for at least an hour or until the physician gives orders otherwise. Strangely, some persons become excited after they regain consciousness from an electric shock and do themselves permanent or even fatal damage by trying to walk around.

See also the item BURNS BY ELECTRIC CURRENT on pages 372, 373 of this same chapter.

## SMOKE INHALATION

A major hazard of firefighting is the damage caused by the breathing of smoke. News items relating to fires frequently mention the number of people who suffer from smoke inhalation without giving details on the seriousness of the condition.

Smoke from burning buildings has become progressively more noxious in recent years due to the use of plastics and synthetics, both in building structures and in furnishings. Smoke from burning buildings now contains many irritating gases which do actual damage to the tissue of the lungs and the air passages. The symptoms of smoke inhalation consist largely of difficulty in breathing. The problem may develop immediately or may be delayed for as long as two days. Carbon monoxide

411

E
M
E
R
G
E
N
C
I
E
S

poisoning is also common in such cases. In severe cases pulmonary edema and/or bacterial pneumonia may develop. Persons who have inhaled smoke should be observed for at least two days even though they exhibit no immediate symptoms.

### What to Do

The essential consideration in treating a person who has inhaled smoke is to maintain an adequate source of air or oxygen. As his breathing becomes handicapped, he may not receive as much oxygen as his body demands. Wafting a stream of oxygen beneath his nostrils is helpful. The attending doctor may order medication to reduce the swelling of tissues lining the patient's air passages. In extreme cases, a mechanical respirator may be necessary.

## SPINAL CORD INJURIES

The spinal cord is the downward continuation of the brain. Many of the nerves that supply the various parts of the body both for sensation and for motor control are attached directly to the spinal cord and emerge between the vertebrae. Violent accidents pose the danger that vertebrae of the back or of the neck may have been broken and the spinal cord injured.

The structure of the spinal cord resembles that of the brain rather than that of the nerves. When the spinal cord is pinched or severed, all of the nerves below the level of injury are forever after useless, and the muscles that these nerves supplied can no longer be controlled by the brain. Paraplegia, in which the victim's legs are paralyzed, is the result of a severing of the spinal cord in the upper part of the back.

### What to Do

For the first-aid handling of injuries in which the spinal cord may have been damaged, see the item FRACTURES OF BONES on pages 392, 393 of this same chapter, and the item SPINAL INJURIES in chapter 4, volume 3.

## SPORTS INJURIES

Understandably these injuries continue to increase as the population's participation in sports increases. The greatest increase in sports participation in recent years has been in the unsupervised sports, such as skiing.

### What to Do

For instruction on the first-aid handling of injuries that may result from participation in sports, see the General Index under such headings as Bandaging Methods; Dislocation; Diving, Related Emergencies; Drowning; Fractures; Injury, Severe; Sprain; and Strains.

## SPRAINS

For a definition and description of sprains, see chapter 21, volume 2. The joints most commonly sprained are the ankle, the knee, and the wrist.

### What to Do

It is advisable that a physician examine a sprained joint for any possible associated fractures. The physician will also advise on how long the patient should avoid using the sprained joint.

1. Immediately following the injury in which a joint is sprained, the application of a cravat bandage to support the joint helps to relieve the patient's discomfort. For the method of applying such a bandage, see pages 359-361 in this same chapter. A cravat bandage should not be left in place for long, however, because of a tendency for swelling in the vicinity of the injured joint that would make the cravat bandage too tight.

2. While a sprained joint continues to be swollen (which may be a few hours or even several days), it should be supported by an elastic bandage which allows for a reasonable amount of swelling. This bandage should be applied firmly but not so tightly as to interfere with the circulation of blood.

3. Once the tendency to swelling has ceased, a firmer support may be

applied, such as a strapping of adhesive tape. This should be applied by someone who has been trained in the use of adhesive bandages. Otherwise, the patient's blood circulation might be endangered.

4. During the first one to three days after the injury, or while a tendency for the joint to swell still persists, an ice bag can be applied to the injured joint. This tends to relieve pain and reduce swelling. The ice bag should be covered with a cloth so as not to come in direct contact with the skin.

5. Once the tendency to swelling has ceased, heat should be applied rather than cold. This increases the circulation of blood through the injured tissues and thus hastens healing.

6. For a sprained wrist, the forearm and hand should be carried in a sling. For a sprained knee or ankle, the patient should be kept in bed for the first day or two or until he can walk with crutches. Even then, the injured part should be supported in a horizontal position for at least fifteen minutes out of each hour.

## STINGS
A. STINGS BY BEES, HORNETS, WASPS, AND YELLOW JACKETS
B. STINGS BY MARINE ANIMALS
C. STINGS BY SCORPIONS

A. *Stings by Bees, Hornets, Wasps, and Yellow Jackets.* Usually these stings are relatively harmless even though they produce painful swelling, redness, and itching at the site of the sting. Several stings at the same time, however, may inject sufficient venom into the victim's tissues to make him quite ill.

The serious fact in connection with stings by bees, hornets, wasps, and yellow jackets is that a few persons are sensitive to the toxins injected by these insects to the extent that anaphylactic shock develops. In such cases we deal with a life-threatening situation.

1. For those occasional cases in which anaphylactic shock develops, see page 409 of this same chapter for the method of emergency treatment.

2. In the usual case of a bee sting, the first procedure is to remove the stinger which includes the venom sac that the bee has deposited in the skin of the victim. Don't pull it out by grasping it with fingernails or tweezers, for thus you may squeeze more venom into the tissues. Try instead to scrape the stinger off gently with an object such as a knife blade, or loosen it with a needle so that you can remove it by sideways motion. Hornets and wasps do not leave a stinger in the skin. They are able to sting repeatedly.

The sting of a honeybee produces an allergic reaction characterized by swelling, redness, and itching. (Note stinger of honeybee left in center of affected area.)

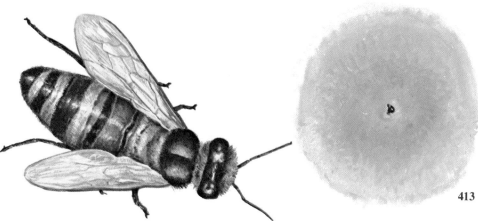

413

**3. Place an adhesive bandage over the site of the sting and soak this with a strong solution of Epsom salts.**

B. *Stings by Marine Animals.*

1. *Catfish.* The saltwater catfish has a barbed stinger at the base of its large dorsal fin, the barb being strong enough to penetrate shoe leather. Accidents usually occur when a fisherman attempts to remove the catfish from a hook, the sting, of course, being inflicted on the hand. The principal dangers are possible allergic reaction or infection.

### What to Do

**Treat the sting of a catfish the same as a snakebite. There is no antivenin available. See the item *Snakebite* on pages 362-365 of this same chapter.**

2. *Jellyfish.* The sting of the jellyfish is inflicted by long tentacles, usually on the victim's leg. The sting causes a feeling of illness which may last for several hours. An allergic reaction occurs in an occasional case.

### What to Do

**Treatment consists of soaking the affected foot and leg in diluted ammonia water (about 4 oz. [120 ml.] to a gallon [4 liters] of water). After soaking it from ten to fifteen minutes in the diluted ammonia water, soak it in hot water to which Epsom salts has been added (6 ounces [180 gm.] to a gallon [4 liters] of water). This tends to relieve the pain. After the soaks, the part should be kept slightly elevated above the level of the body. If the glands in the groin become painful, an ice bag should be applied here for about 20 minutes out of each hour.**

3. *Stingrays.* When a stingray is accidentally stepped on, its whiplike tail can inflict a painful lash, the stinger being located near the base of the animal's tail. The sting produces a painful swelling of the leg. The area may become black and blue, and serious infection may develop. Damage is caused both by the injection of venom and by the injury to the tissues, with possibility of infection.

### What to Do

**1. Spread the wound open and wash it thoroughly with cold water.**

**2. Apply a firm bandage around the leg, as for snakebite, about two inches above the injury. Do this as soon as possible and make it firm enough to retard the spread of the poison through the superficial tissues but not so firm as to obstruct the flow of blood in the deep vessels. It should be possible to place one's finger beneath the bandage after it has been fastened in place.**

**3. Remove any remains of the stinger that may be still within the wound.**

**4. Arrange a hot bath for the injured leg, continuing it for as long as one hour or more and adding hot water as necessary to keep the temperature as high as the victim can reasonably tolerate. This helps to destroy the venom.**

**5. It is advisable to have a physician examine the wound in case it needs to be sutured and in case the victim may benefit by antibiotics to combat the infection.**

C. *Stings by Scorpions.* Two species of scorpions frequent the southwestern states, the stings of which are serious but not usually fatal. The stings of scorpions in Africa and Asia are more serious and often fatal. The situation is most serious in the case of a child; the younger the child, the greater the danger of death.

### What to Do

**Antivenin prepared especially for scorpion stings is the only satisfactory treatment. A doctor should be contacted at once to see if antivenin is available. Otherwise, keeping the patient quiet and warm are the important things. The patient may experience dizziness, vomiting, increased production of saliva, and even shock.**

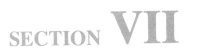

SECTION **VII**

# Home
# Treatments

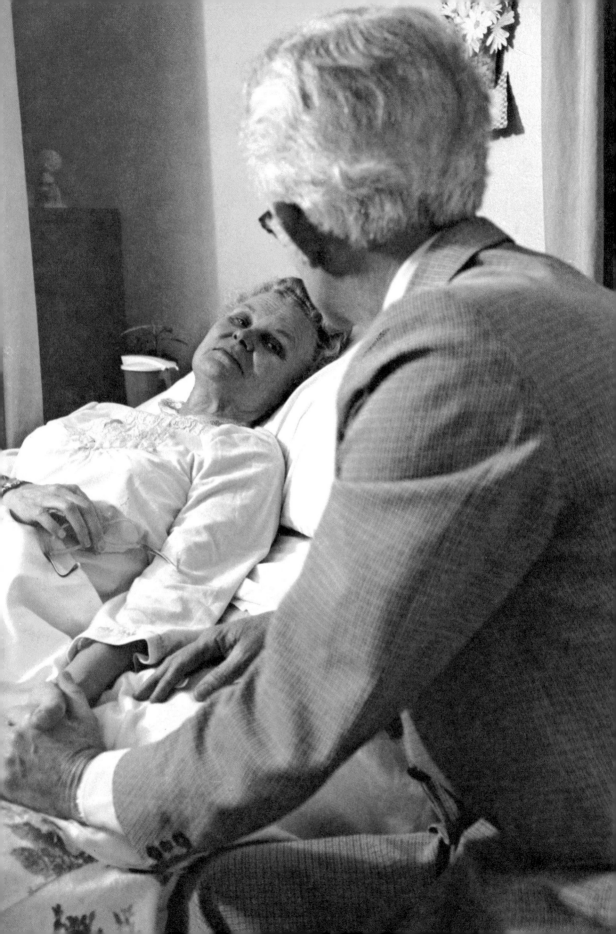

# *When Someone in Your Home Is Ill*

In many cases it is best for a seriously ill person to be cared for in a hospital. There facilities for precise diagnosis are provided. On the other hand, there are times when it is desirable instead to care for an ill person at home, such as following a stay in the hospital. Home care can even have its advantages. The patient benefits by being spared the bustle of a hospital and profits by the loving care and close attention that relatives can give.

This chapter deals with the patient partially or completely confined to bed at home. It is generally assumed that the patient is not to be up and out of bed because of the seriousness of his condition. It should be emphasized, however, that for most patients confined to bed, getting up and around is most important in the period of convalescence. To what extent such activity should be encouraged depends upon the medical condition of the patient, and of course in most cases upon consultation with the patient's physician. At first, and particularly with partially paralyzed patients, care should be given to prevent falling. Sometimes it is necessary to insist that the patient not get up unless someone stands by. Many of the principles and instructions given in this chapter apply during the period of convalescence.

The essence of care for a sick person is to place him in circumstances most favorable for his rehabilitation. By rehabilitation we generally mean one of three things: (1) return to the patient's usual way of life; (2) adoption of a way of life which eliminates the conditions that have caused his present illness—an improved pattern of living; or (3) development of a satisfying life program which makes allowance for the persisting limitations that his illness has caused and yet enables him to live productively.

Rehabilitation occurs gradually. It involves the process of healing: the restoration of torn tissues, the mending of a broken bone, or the development of immunity to an infection. And because of delay in the process, the patient faces the hazard of discouragement or even depression. It is here that the family environment is particularly helpful. Being part of the family group, engaging by proxy in the activities of family members, receiving the love and encouragement of dear ones—these often contribute more to rehabilitation than do medicines or counsel sessions.

Home care for a sick person does not

423

replace professional supervision; it complements it. Depending on the nature of the patient's illness, there may be need for supervision, not only by the physician, but also by other qualified health professionals. The visiting nurse, the physical therapist, the occupational therapist, the speech therapist, the psychologist, the social service worker, the vocational counselor, the chaplain—any one or more of these may be needed in a given case. The family members most involved in the care of the patient must work in close cooperation with these professionals.

The patient being cared for at home must be taught and encouraged to share in the responsibility for his rehabilitation. He should not be allowed to become content to let others wait on him. He must do as much for himself as his condition permits. Only as he learns to be independent and to function in his own right, can his recovery be complete.

### The Home Environment

The room in which a sick person lives and receives care has much to do with his comfort and speed of recovery. Some homes are arranged more favorably than others for the care of a sick person. Thus the exact arrangement will have to be adapted to the individual case.

Ideally, the room chosen should be pleasantly decorated, should admit sunlight when desired, should have provision for heating and cooling as needed, should provide ventilation without causing a draft, and should be near a bathroom or toilet. The room should be clean and in order, each needed article kept in its designated place. Food should not be kept in the room, and all used dishes and soiled linen should be removed promptly after use. A potted plant or a few flowers may be permissible, but none with a strong odor.

The room should be aired once or twice a day, even in cold weather, by opening wide the doors and windows. At such times the patient should be well covered, if in bed, or should wear adequate clothing if sitting up or walk-

**Choice of a home sickroom must take into account factors such as ventilation, sunlight, and bathroom facilities.**

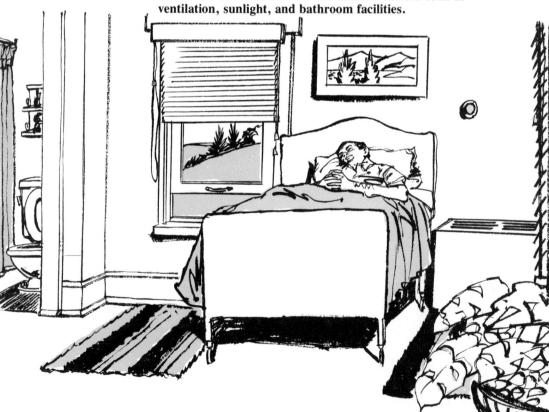

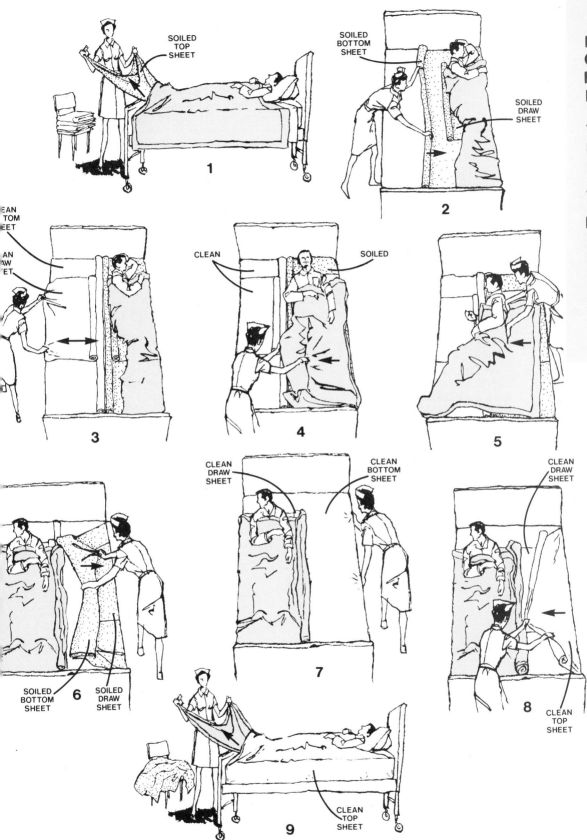

1

SOILED TOP SHEET

2

SOILED BOTTOM SHEET

SOILED DRAW SHEET

3

CLEAN BOTTOM SHEET

CLEAN DRAW SHEET

4

CLEAN

SOILED

5

6

SOILED BOTTOM SHEET

SOILED DRAW SHEET

7

CLEAN DRAW SHEET

CLEAN BOTTOM SHEET

8

CLEAN DRAW SHEET

CLEAN TOP SHEET

9

CLEAN TOP SHEET

427

**Procedure for changing sheets when patient cannot be moved from the bed. See description in this chapter for details to be followed in the progressive steps here illustrated.**

Lift the patient's feet, with knees flexed, over the closely rolled bedding, and, going to the other side of the bed, gently turn the patient back over the rolled sheets onto the fresh, smoothed portion, keeping the covering blanket in place (5). Then quickly remove the soiled bedding and draw the fresh bedding into place on this second half of the bed and tuck it in snuggly all around (6, 7). Place the clean top sheet over the blanket, and then, holding the sheet in place, slide the blanket out from under the sheet and lay it on top of this upper sheet (8, 9). If a second blanket is to be used, it can now be placed on the first one. Arrange the bedspread as before directed and tuck all in at the foot, being careful not to cause discomfort by drawing the bedding too tight over the patient's feet.

The patient can make use of several pillows of various sizes to add wonderfully to his comfort. They make comfortable positions possible by lessening the muscular tension. For example, when the patient is lying on his back with his knees flexed, a pillow under the knees and another for the feet to rest against are helpful. A weak or helpless patient turned on one side appreciates a pillow tucked against his back to support it, and a tiny pillow slipped under the abdomen helps. When the patient is lying on his side, flexing the upper knee a little more than the under one and placing a pillow between his knees is restful and relaxing. When the patient is able to sit up in bed, a kitchen chair nicely serves the purpose of a back support. Turn it upside down with the legs against the head of the bed so that the back forms an inclining plane (see accompanying illustration). Pad it well with pillows. (When a regular hospital bed can be obtained, this improvisation is unnecessary.)

If the patient is weak, a pillow under each arm while he is sitting up in bed makes him more comfortable; and, again, pillows as knee supports and foot rests are useful. One must be careful, however, in making a patient com-

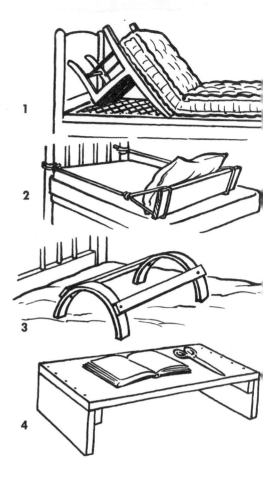

Types of bed-comfort aids: 1. Improvised back support. 2. Cushioned footrest. 3. Cradle to hold bedclothing off sensitive surfaces. 4. Portable worktable. Below: closeup of footrest.

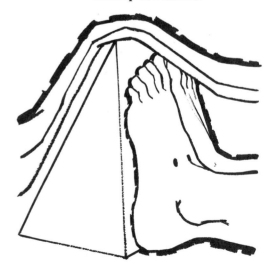

ber may be given as a medicine and thus provide a physiologic laxative.

### How to Give an Enema

Occasionally it may be necessary to give an enema to avoid severe constipation. Whenever possible, the patient should be encouraged to use the bathroom or a commode as the enema is given. Chemical enemas are convenient and require a minimum of time and effort. These are conveniently packaged and available at any drugstore. The substance contained in a tube is injected into the rectum, and this has the effect of stimulating bowel action.

For those who wish to use a water enema to meet the needs of a bed patient, a certain amount of equipment must be available. The bed should be protected by means of a plastic sheet covered with a large towel. Have the patient lying on his back with the knees flexed. The patient's gown should be raised above the hips as one rim of a bedpan is placed under the patient's hips in a way that allows the open portion to protrude toward the patient's heels. After placing the bedpan, the patient's back should be supported with a pillow. A newspaper spread over the patient's knees and legs forms a protection to the upper sheet should the water be expelled with force.

Bring to the bedside a roll of toilet tissue, vaseline, a plastic bucket, and an enema can or enema bag holding the solution to be injected. The solution should be warm—about 100° F. (38° C.) unless otherwise ordered by the doctor. A saline enema (about two teaspoons of table salt per quart of water) is preferable in most cases. Any other type of enema should be ordered by a doctor. To avoid too great force in the injection, the enema can or bag should be no more than two or three feet above the level of the patient's hips.

The solution is allowed to flow into the patient's rectum at a moderate rate. If the patient has a desire to expel the solution as soon as the enema is begun, stop the flow for a minute, lower the can or bag, and begin again slowly. Better results are obtained if the solution can be retained for a few minutes and then expelled gradually. An adult patient should be able to retain one or two quarts of the enema solution. The injection may need to be repeated if good results are not secured with the first injection. Always lift the patient's hips with one hand before removing the bedpan, as the skin easily adheres to it. The bedpan should be covered immediately when removed and emptied without delay.

Special attention should be given to the cleansing of the skin about the rectum after a bowel movement. The use of toilet paper alone may not be sufficient. It is important to keep the area clean and dry to prevent skin damage or irritation.

The bedpan may be used for ordinary bowel movements and for emptying the bladder in women patients. It should be remembered, however, that lying over a bedpan for a bowel movement or even for emptying the bladder is an abnormal position for these functions. Often more straining and work is required than in the normal sitting position over the toilet seat or over a bedside commode.

### Showering or Bathing

Unless a patient is unable to leave his bed, he should be encouraged to shower daily. This routine gets him out of bed, provides exercise and relief from lying, and is simple and easy. A stool may be placed in the shower so the patient can sit while showering, if necessary. If the patient can be helped in and out of a bathtub, bathing may even be preferred to showering. The patient's bed may be made while he is in the tub.

A bed patient should have a bath of some sort every day, and a soap bath at least every other day. A plain sponge bath of warm or cool water may be given on alternate days. A description detailing the procedure for bathing a bed patient follows:

H
O
M
E

T
R
E
A
T
M
E
N
T
S

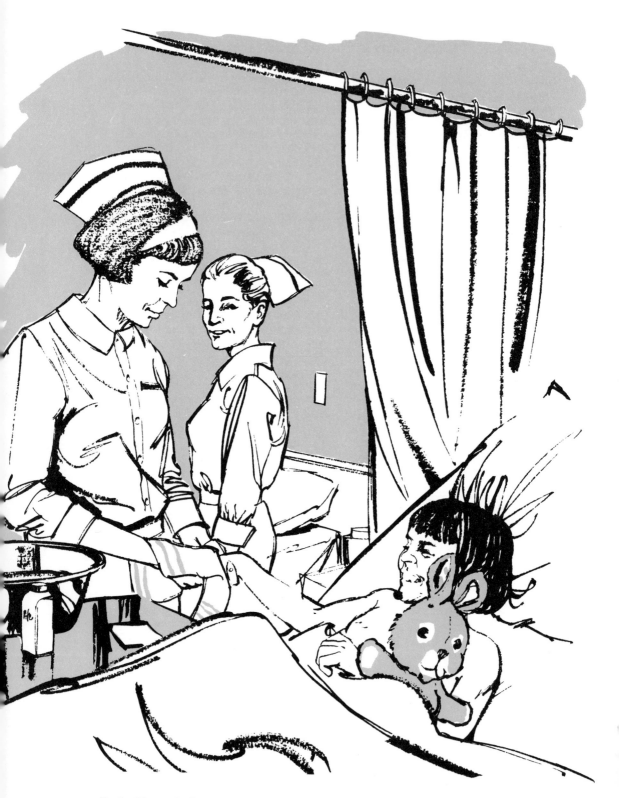

In bathing a bed patient the procedure begins with the face, neck, and `ears, and progresses to the arms and hands, each part being thoroughly dried in turn.

skin pads are very helpful.

The following counsel on care of patients in the home, published years ago, has an up-to-date ring and provides an excellent summary:

"Those who minister to the sick should understand the importance of careful attention to the laws of health. Nowhere is obedience to these laws more important than in the sickroom. Nowhere does so much depend upon faithfulness in little things on the part of the attendants. In cases of serious illness, a little neglect, a slight inattention to a patient's special needs or dangers, the manifestation of fear, excitement, or petulance, even a lack of sympathy, may turn the scale that is balancing life and death, and cause to go down to the grave a patient who otherwise might have recovered.

"The efficiency of the nurse depends, to a great degree, upon physical vigor. The better the health, the better will she be able to endure the strain of attendance upon the sick, and the more successfully can she perform her duties. Those who care for the sick should give special attention to diet, cleanliness, fresh air, and exercise. . . .

"Where the illness is serious, requiring the attendance of a nurse night and day, the work should be shared by at least two efficient nurses, so that each may have opportunity for rest and for exercise in the open air. . . .

"Nurses, and all who have to do with the sickroom, should be cheerful, calm, and self-possessed. All hurry, excitement, or confusion, should be avoided. Doors should be opened and shut with care, and the whole household be kept quiet. In cases of fever, special care is needed when the crisis comes and the fever is passing away. Then constant watching is often necessary. Igno-

rance, forgetfulness, and recklessness have caused the death of many who might have lived had they received proper care from judicious, thoughtful nurses."—E. G. White, *The Ministry of Healing,* pp. 219-222.

Anticipating the possible need of having to care for a sick relative in the home or even in preparation for a specific need, it is recommended that advantage be taken of courses offered in home nursing by the American Red Cross or other community or church agencies. Really almost every homemaker will become a home nurse sometime. In any specific problem, help is available from community agencies such as the Public Health Department, the Visiting Nurses' Association, or homecare facilities associated with medical centers.

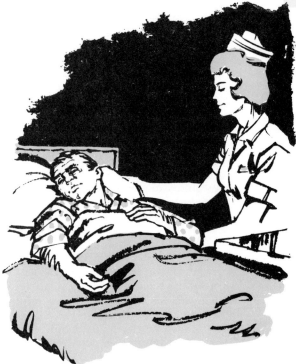

439

# Simple Home Treatments

It is inconceivable that every slight ache or pain be reason for calling a doctor. Such a practice would result in an impossible situation. It is reasonable that people use domestic remedies for relief from obviously minor symptoms. Actually such a practice is encouraged by the medical profession. But medical help should certainly be sought when a symptom is severe, when it persists, when it returns frequently, or when any doubt arises as to its significance. Such symptoms should be considered as warning signals of an abnormality that needs professional attention.

The knowledge and practice of healthful living habits will do much in preventing disease conditions with their unpleasant symptoms. It is best to eat the apple a day that keeps the doctor away. One of the main objectives of these three volumes is to acquaint the reader with the principles of healthful living and thus to minimize the necessity of treatment of any kind. But illnesses and injuries do occur, and for minor ones every householder should be equipped to administer simple remedies.

Unfortunately, wall cabinets in many homes are stocked with medicines for headache, acid stomach, sleeplessness, et cetera; and members of the family tend to use these rather indiscriminately. Self-medication is encouraged by advertisements on television and radio, in the press, and in the drugstore. People are filling themselves with chemicals that actually cause damage to the body's tissues.

In contrast to medication by drugs, there are available to all, simple treatments which do not leave residuals in the body. These consist of the rational use of natural remedies such as water, light, controlled exercise, and rest. With these remedies, as with the use of drugs, self-treatment should be restricted to only minor symptoms which do not warrant calling for medical help, to temporary emergency situations when waiting for the doctor, or to treatment done under medical direction. The results of these treatments depend on the natural physiological response of the body to its surroundings and to its own activity. It should be understood that any major treatment suggested here should be carried out with the approval of the patient's physician.

## Hydrotherapy

Among the simple drugless methods of treating disease or simple injuries, the use of heat and cold ranks high in importance. Heat or cold may be easily applied with the use of that most common substance, water, in one of its three states—liquid, vapor (steam), and solid (ice). The use of water in treatment is called "hydrotherapy." Only a few of the simplest treatments can be considered here. None of these require hospital equipment. While these simple treatments can be given in the home, careful observation of all details of instruction is necessary, for even these simple treatments wrongly applied may do harm. Usually, anything with potential for good may do harm when wrongly used.

*Characteristic Effects of Heat and Cold.* When one bathes his face with cold water or takes a quick dip or plunges into cold water, after the first shock there comes a delightful feeling of invigoration, with quickened circulation and soon a glow of warmth in the skin. A concomitant result is greater energy for either muscular or brain work, all normal body activities being stimulated. These changes that result from a brief application of cold water to the skin are spoken of as reaction.

People in vigorous health usually react well to cold water, especially after they have become accustomed to its use. The process of becoming accustomed to it may need to be quite gradual, but the health and vigor that result are well worth the time and effort necessary to acquire them, especially in the case of a weakly person.

In treating the sick by the use of hydrotherapy, securing a reaction is important, for upon this depends success in stimulating the activity of the organs not working normally. It may be difficult to secure a good reaction. The patient's circulation may be poor, or he may chill readily. The cold water may have to be applied to only one part of his body at a time, after a hot application has first warmed the skin or while hot applications are being administered to other parts of his body; and the cold application may have to be made with energetic rubbing. In case of chilliness, hot applications sufficient even to produce sweating must be used before a cold application so that the patient will react properly. This is most important and must not be forgotten, especially with such diseases as colds, influenza, and pneumonia.

Internal congestion may be relieved by hot applications over a fairly large skin area as the blood is drawn to the skin surface. This effect results from the attempt of the body to get rid of the heat thus applied. Cold application used for a comparatively long time on a relatively small area of skin will reduce swelling and congestion in the surface area and in the deep structures. The effect on the underlying organs is produced by the nerve connections between specific skin areas and specific organs.

Thus heat alone may be used in treating deep congestions or inflammations, such as lung congestion and pleurisy. The ice bag alone may be used, as with an acute, severely inflamed breast; or, better still, the ice bag may be applied directly over the inflamed part, and hot applications at a distance, as with acute appendicitis—the ice bag over the appendix and hot applications to the legs and feet. Of course, even if appendicitis is suspected the physician should be called. When the head is hot and throbbing, a hot footbath together with cold cloth to the head helps greatly. When the lungs are congested, a hot footbath and very hot fomentations over the congested part draw the blood to the surface and to the feet. An ice bag applied to the chest over the heart, in case of heart disease with a rapid pulse, slows the heartbeat and increases its force. Again, the physician should be called when heart disease is suspected.

Hot applications alternating with cold promptly increase the number of red and white blood cells in active circulation, and a series of such treatments, together with fresh air, sunshine, and nourishing food, are helpful in treating anemia and other diseases of the blood. Alternate hot and cold applications are often beneficial in treating local infection.

441

In giving treatments, seemingly small details are of great importance, and to disregard them may not only nullify the benefit to the patient but actually harm him. Be sure to follow directions carefully. Remember that chilling the patient may cause harm; but, on the other hand, the cold water must be used cold, or little good will be accomplished. Hot applications must be hot, not lukewarm; and mere complaint that they are hot is not sufficient reason for cooling them before they are applied. Burning can be prevented, as will be explained later.

When applying heat, great care must be exercised to avoid damage to a part with poor blood vessels—a point particularly true of the feet. Direct heat application to a part acutely inflamed and swollen should be avoided—direct cold may be much better. The effects of hot and cold water on the body can be clearly demonstrated, but the exact explanation of how these effects take place may not be fully understood. The important thing is that they do occur.

"Heat" and "cold" are comparative terms, and must be defined. This cannot be done with accuracy, since various people differ in their toleration to heat and cold. The temperature sensation produced by water varies according to the condition of the skin, its previous temperature, the vigor of blood circulation, and the season of the year. Testing the temperature of water to be used in hydrotherapy, therefore, should be done with a thermometer as well as with the hand.

*Equipment Needed for Home Hydrotherapy.* Only simple appliances are needed for giving water treatments in the home. Substitutes may be used in emergencies, but it is much better to provide the things listed below:

1. One set of six cloths, wool or half wool, each at least 30 x 36 inches (75 x 90 cm.) in size. An old part-woolen bed blanket cut in four pieces makes four good cloths. These when heated as described in the following procedures are called "fomentations."

2. Two rough friction mitts, without fingers, made from rough toweling or wash cloths.

3. Two hot-water bottles, rubber preferred.

4. One rubber ice bag.

5. One bath thermometer.

6. Two elliptical foot tubs about 16 inches (40 cm.) long and 10 inches (25 cm.) deep.

7. Pans, kettles, towels, sheets, and blankets such as are usually found in the home.

8. Two large, deep metal or plastic cans or buckets. These should be about 12 inches (30 cm.) in diameter and 16 inches (40 cm.) deep.

### Fomentations

A fomentation is a local application of moist heat by means of cloths (largely wool) wrung from boiling water or heated in a steam chest.

*Articles Needed.* Provide a deep dishpan or a large kettle of water to be kept actively boiling, a cover to retain the heat, a set of six fomentation cloths, several Turkish towels, a hand towel, a sheet, a bowl of cold water or ice water, and a table.

*The Patient and the Bed.* See that all clothing is removed so that it doesn't become damp from perspiration. Cover the patient with a sheet plus other covering to keep him warm. See especially that the feet are warm and that they are kept so during the treating. A hot footbath should be given or hot-water bottles put to the feet, this beginning before the fomentations and continuing all the time that the fomentations are being applied.

Protect the bedding by a blanket or sheet folded lengthwise and placed under the patient. After applying the fomentation, cover it with a dry cloth or newspaper in order to protect the bedding above it.

*Preparation of the Fomentation.* If possible, the hot-water kettle and the table should be near the bed, and the preparation of the fomentation should be done quickly so that loss of heat before application will be minimal. Three cloths are necessary for each fomentation if they are to be very hot, one for the dry covering and two to be wrung from boiling water for the inside moist part. If less heat is required, one inside cloth may be sufficient. Two such sets of cloths are necessary so that one fomentation can be in preparation while the other is in use.

Spread out on the table the cloth for the dry covering. Then fold together in three thicknesses the cloth or cloths to be used inside, so as to make a long, narrow piece. Immerse this folded cloth, except the two ends which are held in the hands, in the boiling water. Leave until thoroughly soaked with boiling water, then wring quickly by firm twisting and pulling until water no longer drips from it. If held up by one end, the folded cloth will quickly untwist to its original one-third width. Place this across the middle of the dry fomentation cloth already spread out on the table. Fold the dry ends of the inside cloth over its damp center and then fold the dry outer cloth about the damp inner one. In the folding, the fomentation should be made the right size and shape to fit the part to be treated. It should be large enough to extend slightly beyond the boundaries of this area.

*Procedure.* The fomentation should lie in close contact with the skin and should be renewed in five minutes or less. If necessary, it may be laid over a dry Turkish towel to temper the heat. If unbearably hot, lift the fomentation slightly for a few seconds and rub with the hand the part under it, or remove the moisture on the patient's skin by firm rubbing once or twice with a dry towel wrapped about the hand. Always protect the area being treated from chilling by keeping it covered with a dry fomentation cloth or dry towel when the fomentation is not actually being applied.

To renew the fomentation, prepare another similar one and have it ready to apply immediately upon removing the previous one. At the time of exchange the skin should be dried quickly by using a towel, because moisture remaining on the skin makes it harder for the patient to endure the heat of the newly prepared fomentation.

Unless otherwise directed, three successive applications should be made, covering a period of from ten to fifteen minutes. After the last one is finished, the part should immediately be given a very brief rub with a cold, wet towel or with rubbing alcohol. Dry the skin thoroughly, but quickly, and cover the patient at once to avoid chilling.

*Precautions.* In cases of unconsciousness, paralyzed sensation, diabetes, dropsy, or poor blood vessels, especially in the feet, great care must be taken to avoid burning. The fomentation should be slightly raised at frequent intervals and the hand of the attendant thrust beneath it to test its heat in such cases. This heat testing should be done in as brief a period as possible, however, so as to avoid chilling.

In case of free perspiration, a general cold friction, a wet hand rub, a wet towel rub, or an alcohol rub should be given following the last of the three fomentations.

Apply cold compresses to the head throughout the time of applying fomentations to any other part of the body. In heart disease, usually in high fever, and with a rapid pulse from any cause, an ice bag should be placed over the heart.

In order to relieve pain, the fomentation must be very hot, as hot as can be borne, and should be renewed as soon as it ceases to feel hot. In cases of severe pain, the cold application at the close should be omitted, the treated part being dried and immediately covered with flannel or other dry covering. A test of the efficacy of fomentations is the redness of the skin after completion of the treatment.

If it is not certain that fomentations can be given without chilling the patient, do not give them at all. Moist

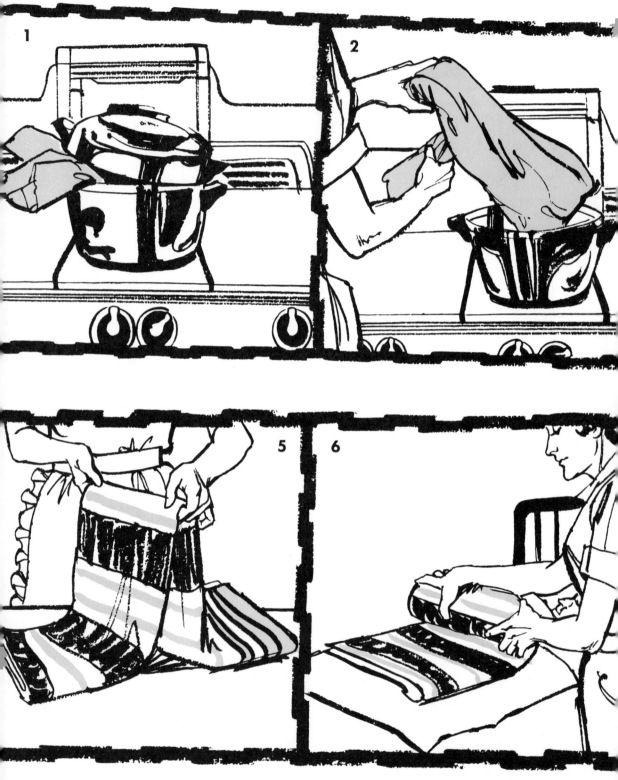

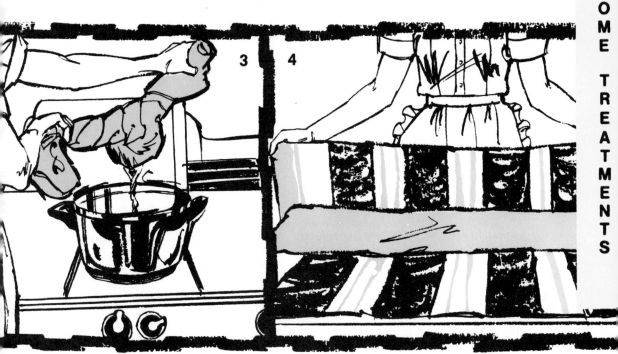

Local treatment by fomentation involves application of moist heat by means of cloths wrung from boiling water, procedure as follows, steps numbered to correspond with numbers on the drawings:

1. Immerse folded cloth to be used inside pack in a pan of boiling water, leaving ends hanging over the edge to be kept dry.

2. Leave until thoroughly soaked; then remove by grasping dry ends.

3. Twist and pull cloth to wring out as much of the water as possible.

4. Hold twisted cloth up by one end to allow it to untwist. Then place it across dry fomentation cloth spread out on the table.

5. Fold the dry outer cloth about the damp inner one to make the pack, which is now ready to be applied to patient.

6. Place fomentation pack in close contact with patient's skin, with a dry towel spread underneath if pack is unbearably hot, and leave it applied for about five minutes.

heat applied by means of a hot-water bottle laid over two thicknesses of moist Turkish toweling is a fair substitute.

*Various Forms.* Applied to the throat and upper chest, fomentations help in relieving sore throat, tonsillitis, cough, bronchitis, lung congestion, et cetera.

When applied to the throat only, the hot cloth should be folded so as to be about eight inches (20 cm.) wide. To protect the lower part of the face, a Turkish towel may be placed across the neck, under the fomentation. The heat pack should be tucked up close below the ears. For the chest only, the fomentation should be folded nearly square

445

and as large as possible. For pleurisy, it should be applied to the side of the chest under the arm, from breastbone to spine; for the kidneys and for lumbago, across the small of the back. For the spine, it should be long and narrow, about six inches (15 cm.) wide. Fomentations to the spine help to promote sleep, and for this purpose they should be only moderately hot. For the knee, the cloth may be folded as for the spine, and, being drawn under the joint, the two ends are wrapped about the front of it, one above the other. The use of two fomentations, one behind and one in front of the knee, at the same time, tucked in snugly to exclude air, may be fully as effective as the single fomentation wrapped around the joint and more comfortable.

Sometimes it is desirable to apply a fomentation to the eye or to some other small area. The full-sized fomentation cloth cannot be used in such cases. A thick pad composed of thirty to fifty layers of gauze, dipped in very hot water and squeezed almost dry, is a good substitute. Since such small fomentations lose heat rapidly, they should be changed every minute or two. Small fomentations are frequently called hot compresses.

Another form of fomentation has been called the revulsive compress, and is given with the following addition: A hand towel is wrung from cold water and spread over the skin surface immediately after the removal of each fomentation. It is pressed firmly against the skin, turned over, again pressed firmly over the skin, and removed. A smooth piece of ice may be rubbed over the skin after each fomentation instead of applying a cold compress. The skin must be quickly wiped dry before heat is again applied.

Alternate hot and cold to the spine, with fomentations as the source of heat, acts as a stimulant and tonic, being used in the case of colds, bronchitis, and similar ailments after the acute stage is past. To the abdomen, it is useful in stimulating the flow of digestive juices and the movements of the stom-ach and bowels. In treating the chest, the abdomen, the neck, or a joint, for the cold part of the treatment use a cloth wrung from cold water rather than a piece of ice.

There are two modifications of the fomentation available commercially. One is the Hydrocollator ®, which consists of material that holds water sewn into pads of convenient size. These pads are heated in a container of water operated electrically and controlled by a thermostat. When taken out of the water these pads will hold heat for a prolonged time; they do not drip water. They should be covered with toweling and applied to the part to be heated. These hot packs have certain advantages because of ease of preparation, but they also have disadvantages, such as not being easily molded to the part being treated, and being heavy.

Another modification of the fomentation available commercially is an electrically heated pad (Thermophore ®), so designed that moisture from the body accumulates during the application and thus simulates the condition of a cloth fomentation. Special precautions must be taken with its use. A special switch which must be actively pressed during the application is a safety feature.

### Local Cold Applications

*Cold Compress.* This is a local application of cold by means of a cloth wrung from cold water. Hand towels or ordinary cotton cloths may be used. These should be folded to the desired size, and wrung from cold water, preferably ice water. The wringing should be barely sufficient to prevent dripping. As a continuous cold application, the compress must be changed frequently, always before it becomes warm to any great extent. The thicker the compress, the less frequently will it require changing. Cold compresses may be applied to the head, the neck, over the heart or the lungs, to the abdomen, the spine, or other parts. (See paragraph at the end of this subsection for conditions in which cold applications may be used.)